K. Sugano (Editor in Chief)
H. Yamamoto, H. Kita (Eds.)

Double-Balloon Endoscopy

Theory and Practice

K. Sugano (Editor in Chief)
H. Yamamoto, H. Kita (Eds.)

Double-Balloon Endoscopy

Theory and Practice

With 109 Figures, Mostly in Color

Springer

Kentaro Sugano, M.D., Ph.D.
Professor, Department of Internal Medicine
Division of Gastroenterology, Jichi Medical University
3311-1 Yakushiji, Shimotsuke, Tochigi 329-0498, Japan

Hironori Yamamoto, M.D., Ph.D.
Associate Professor, Department of Internal Medicine
Division of Gastroenterology, Jichi Medical University
3311-1 Yakushiji, Shimotsuke, Tochigi 329-0498, Japan

Hiroto Kita, M.D., Ph.D.
Assistant Professor, Department of Internal Medicine
Division of Gastroenterology, Jichi Medical University
3311-1 Yakushiji, Shimotsuke, Tochigi 329-0498, Japan

ISBN 978-4-431-56089-0 ISBN 978-4-431-34205-2 (eBook)
DOI 10.1007/978-4-431-34205-2
Springer-Verlag Tokyo Berlin Heidelberg New York
Printed on acid-free paper

Springer is a part of Springer Science+Business Media
springer.com

Softcover reprint of the hardcover 1st edition 2006

This English translation is based on the Japanese original
K. Sugano, H. Yamamoto, H. Kita: Double-Balloon Endoscopy
Published by Nankodo Co., Ltd.

Typesetting, printing and binding: Kato Bunmeisha, Japan

Preface

The double-balloon endoscope came about as the combined result of a brilliant idea and tenacious effort by Hironori Yamamoto, an associate professor in our department. The first clinical application of the double-balloon method was made for diagnosis of hemangioma in the small intestine of a patient with Maffucci's syndrome, as described in this book. Dr. Yamamoto attached a handmade balloon to an upper gastrointestinal endoscope and manually inflated and deflated the balloon, with a sphygmomanometer monitoring the pressure. The maneuverability and the time required for examination appeared to be similar to those in the procedure using a conventional enteroscope, although I was impressed by the fact that double-balloon endoscopy actually revealed hemangioma previously suspected by contrast radiogram, validating the concept of the double-balloon method. However, there were various problems with the handmade device, including balloon damage, dropout, and air leakage, as well as the patience required on the part of the assistant doctors, all of which made its practical application difficult. Despite these circumstances, Dr. Yamamoto clearly identified and solved the problems one by one. As he describes in chapter 1 of this book, the cooperation of manufacturers such as Nisco and Fujinon was a great help, and many medical staff in our department who continuously assisted him in time-consuming examinations also contributed significantly to the practical application of this novel modality of endoscopy. Through the development of this procedure, we directly observed many previously unrecognized lesions and performed endoscopic treatments that had been possible only by surgical operation, and we found that the procedure was tremendously useful for a variety of disorders. Now the double-balloon endoscopy system distributed by Fujinon is in clinical use worldwide and contributes to the diagnosis and treatment of disorders in the small intestine and other regions of the gastrointestinal tract that were not easily accessible by conventional approaches. However, there was no guidebook for systematic training in this procedure, and we believed it was important to provide an opportunity for many clinicians to learn the procedure and perform it properly; thus we decided to publish this book. Consequently, the book provides a range of techniques and tips developed through trial and error by Dr. Yamamoto and our colleagues, who are co-authors of the book. A DVD is included to provide a visual presentation of specific manipulations.

As described in the book, the double-balloon method was initially intended for use in enteroscopy; however, the double-balloon endoscope allows observation of the entire gastrointestinal tract, including the stomach and the large intestine. In addition, the endoscope allows shortening and straightening of the intestinal tract and is suitable for examination of a reconstituted intestine after Roux-en-Y anastomosis and colonoscopy in which insertion is difficult. Thus, we have changed the initially planned title *Double-Balloon Enteroscopy* to *Double-Balloon Endoscopy*.

Some people were skeptical of the clinical significance of the procedure, because intestinal diseases were previously considered to be uncommon and the development of the double-balloon endoscope paralleled that of the capsule endoscope. As evidenced by our short-term experience described in this book, however, we realized that a variety of lesions, hitherto unrecognized because of their limited accessibility, were present in the small intestine as well as in the blind loop. Compared with the capsule endoscope, the double-balloon endoscope produces images with much higher resolution, provides maneuverability that allows retrograde examination, and permits concomitant use of a variety of diagnostic techniques such as biopsy, dye spraying, and contrast-enhanced examination. It should also be noted that the double-balloon endoscope is compatible with almost all procedures for endoscopic treatment. In combination with those procedures, double-balloon endoscopy now appears to be far superior to capsule endoscopy with respect to diagnostic and therapeutic performance.

This book is intended to be useful as a technical manual and does not include details of individual diseases and the basis for their diagnosis. It may be somewhat difficult for complete novices to understand the initial settings and other technical details that we are accustomed to. In the future, we will make revisions in response to questions and criticisms from readers. We hope, however, that the book will contribute to the elucidation of the pathophysiological mechanisms of intestinal diseases and their treatments, which we believe will evolve dramatically in the twenty-first century with the general availability of double-balloon endoscopy.

Kentaro Sugano
Department of Internal Medicine
Division of Gastroenterology
Jichi Medical University, Japan
January 2006

Contents

List of Editors and Authors

Editor in Chief

Kentaro Sugano — Professor
Department of Gastroenterology, Jichi Medical University

Editors

Hironori Yamamoto — Associate Professor
Department of Gastroenterology, Jichi Medical University

Hiroto Kita — Assistant Professor
Department of Gastroenterology, Jichi Medical University

Authors

Hironori Yamamoto — Associate Professor
Department of Gastroenterology, Jichi Medical University

Masayuki Takano — Fujinon Corporation

Syuuichi Yamataka — Fujinon Corporation

Tomohiko Miyata — Department of Gastroenterology, Jichi Medical University

Yutaka Sekine — Internal Medicine, Nasu Minami Hospital

Tomonori Yano — Department of Gastroenterology, Jichi Medical University

Keijiro Sunada — Department of Gastroenterology, Jichi Medical University

Yoshikazu Hayashi — Department of Gastroenterology, Jichi Medical University

Hiroyuki Sato — Department of Gastroenterology, Jichi Medical University

Toshihiko Higashizawa — Department of Gastroenterology, Jichi Medical University

Michiko Iwamoto — Department of Gastroenterology, Jichi Medical University

Hiroto Kita — Department of Gastroenterology, Jichi Medical University

Contents of Attachment DVD

The DVD that comes with this book, *Procedure Manual for Inserting the Double-Ballon Endoscope*, was provided by Fujinon Corporation. Contents are as follows.

1. Introduction — Introduction of the products, preparation, explanation of operation
2. Clinical Examples — How to operate the products
3. Interviews — Interviews with Dr. Hironori Yamamoto

DVD Planning and creative work : Fujinon Corporation

DVD VIDEO	Stereo sound track recorded on Sony Linear PCM		Image size 4 : 3
	Time : 36 min.	Color	
	Single-sided single layer	MPEG2	

1 What Is a Double-Balloon Endoscope?

The double-balloon endoscope is an endoscope that is used in a novel insertion method developed to ensure smooth insertion into the distal small intestine. Its principle came to my mind in 1997. I was involved in community health care after graduating from Jichi Medical University and was not familiar with endoscopic expertise, such as enteroscopy, until I went back to my alma mater 11 years after graduation. My thoughts resulted in a novel idea. In community health care settings, the lack of advice from instructors often required ingenuity to solve problems. Over the 10 years following graduation, I developed critical thinking skills instead of being content with the status quo.

To be honest, I thought enteroscopy was an awful examination when I first witnessed an enteroscopic examination. During push enteroscopy, a long endoscope was inserted through the mouth while the patient complained of discomfort. On the fluoroscopic monitor, I found the endoscope forming a loop, stretching the intestine, but advancing little. Efforts to advance the endoscope farther made it form a larger loop with the tip stalled, which caused more discomfort to the patient. Despite the prolonged examination, the endoscope tip reached only 50 cm distal to the ligament of Treitz, and the examination was discontinued with no elucidation of pathologic conditions.

The examination left a deep impression on me, and I wondered why the endoscope had not advanced despite such an effort. A few days later, while driving, I was still wondering and suddenly realized that stretching the intestine prevents insertion. It was well known at the time that straightening the intestinal tract helped insertion of a colonoscope, and a semi-rigid overtube was used to prevent the straightened intestine from forming a loop again. Such an overtube was also used with a push enteroscope, but it was very difficult to straighten an intricately curved small intestine. Thus, my new idea was not to straighten the intestine but to use a balloon-attached flexible overtube to prevent stretching the curved intestine. Furthermore, another balloon was attached to the endoscope tip to prevent the deeply inserted endoscope from slipping out while advancing the overtube — and a prototype of the double-balloon endoscope was thus developed.

The double-balloon endoscope is often described as a type of "measuring worm" and the procedure as achieving "with balloon support, shortening the intestine and endoscope insertion." Each description is close to but not exactly the same as my concept. The primary objective is to prevent stretching the intestine. The intestine is shortened only to make the best use of the working length of the endoscope and facilitate its insertion. Accordingly, I believed from the beginning that this approach would be useful in colonoscopy as well, especially in patients with adhesions, which make insertion of a colonoscope difficult.

I asked endoscope manufacturers for their cooperation as soon as the principle of insertion occurred to me, but they turned me down. They had convincing reasons, and it could not be helped. However, it was good not to abandon my idea. They told me that the principle was merely an armchair theory and unlikely to be substantiated in the clinical setting; moreover, the endoscope, if practicable, would be unprofitable from the viewpoint of the enteroscope market.

Because endoscope manufacturers declined to cooperate, I had no choice but to do it myself. A balloon was attached to the tip of a plastic tube purchased at a hardware store and this concoction was used in combination with an endoscope. Because of the lack of an air route for the balloon at the endoscope tip, it was attached in a retrograde direction so the air route came out the forceps channel (Fig. 1.1). I could not test the initial prototype clinically and asked Dr. Yukihiro Sato, one of my fellows, for cooperation. He willingly agreed to be a study volunteer. The first trial was conducted with a prototype overtube that had an outer diameter of 14 mm. The volunteer was given pharyngeal anesthesia only, without sedation, and the procedure was not tolerated because the vomiting reflex manifested before the tube reached the small intestine, failing to test the principle. Next, we took turns being the operator and the study volunteer, and the procedure was tested on me. I was unable to tolerate the examination either and gave it up.

I therefore concluded that the safety and usefulness should be demonstrated in animal studies before clinical application, so I tested the procedure in dogs. The procedure was then approved by our institutional ethics committee and used in the clinical setting.

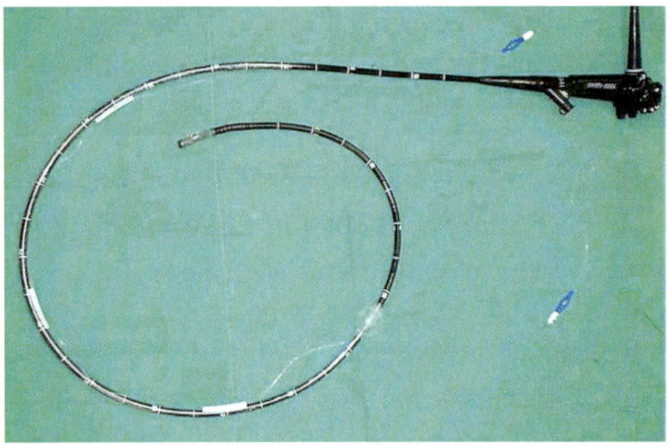

Fig. 1.1. Prototype double-balloon endoscope equipped with a hand-made balloon-attached overtube

The first three patients were examined with an upper endoscope that had an outer diameter of 7.7 mm and a working length of 103 cm together with a balloon-attached overtube with an outer diameter of 12 mm and a length of 75 cm. The fourth patient was examined with an enteroscope with a working length of 200 cm in combination with a 140-cm overtube. All examinations were successful; and total enteroscopy was completed with the endoscope tip advanced into the large intestine in the fourth patient. The results were reported at scientific meetings in Japan and other countries and published in *Gastrointestinal Endoscopy* [1].

A few questions remained concerning the clinical safety and effectiveness of this method. One was whether the balloon would grip the less robust small intestine safely and adequately without patient discomfort; thus, an endoscope was inserted with the supporting point as a fulcrum. I believed that appropriate selection of balloon materials, pressure that ensured a wide margin of safety, and a soft balloon with lower pressure and a larger contact area would provide a satisfactory grip. The luminal diameter of the small intestine varies among individuals, and the diameter differs between the jejunum and the ileum. Moreover, some regions are dilated in response to stenosis; and conditions are, of course, totally different in the large intestine. With these factors taken into consideration, inflation of the balloon was specified in terms of inflation pressure, not air content. This approach allowed a balloon to grip intestinal tracts that have different luminal diameters with the same intensity. To demonstrate the safety and determine the optimal pressure, the following experiment was performed in the small intestine of dogs.

Laparotomy was performed under general anesthesia. A silicon or latex balloon attached to the tip of a rod, with a diameter of 10 mm and an approximate length of 15 cm, was inserted from an incision made in the jejunum to investigate the relation between inflation pressure and resistance to withdrawal.

1. The relation between inflation pressure and grip was measured with two types of balloon (Table 1.1; grip 1 and grip 2 represent two measurements).
2. Withdrawal of the latex balloon with an inflation pressure of 100 mm Hg produced no gross mucosal damage.

These results suggested that a soft latex balloon with an inflation pressure of 40–100 mm Hg was suitable for enteroscopy, and the minimum required pressure was determined to be 45 mm Hg.

Table 1.1. Relation between inflation pressure and grip measured with two types of balloon

Balloon pressure (mm Hg)	Grip 1 (g)	Grip 2 (g)
Latex balloon (made from condoms)		
0	0	0
10	0	0
20	20	0
30	30	20
40	70	20
50	80	70
60	120	70
70	200	80
80	200	120
90	220	180
100	100	140
120	180	
140	210	
160	500	
Silicon balloon		
0	0	0
10	0	0
20	0	10
30	10	0
40	10	0
50	20	20
60	20	20
70	20	20
80	20	20
90	20	20
100	20	20
120	30	30
140	60	30
160	60	40
180	60	60
200	80	70
240	360	

Another concern was friction between the overtube and the endoscope. Controlling an endoscope through a long overtube requires eliminating any influence of friction, thereby allowing the endoscope to slide smoothly, even through a curved overtube. The handmade overtube was therefore equipped with a lubricant inlet around one-third the distance from the tip of the overtube so olive oil could be applied during the examination. Currently, the overtube distributed by Fujinon has a convenient internal and external hydrophilic coating by which water injection alone ensures smooth sliding.

Initially, a syringe was used to inflate and deflate a balloon while the internal pressure was being measured with a sphygmomanometer. For marketed devices, a balloon pump controller allows accurate monitoring of the balloon pressure and automatic inflation and deflation of the balloon with the touch of a button, which reduces the time required for the examination.

Tsuneo Nishiguchi, the president of Nisco, cooperated to an extraordinary extent in developing the double-balloon endoscope. Prototypes of a balloon-attached overtube, a balloon at the endoscope tip, and a balloon pump controller were made in cooperation with Nishiguchi. He introduced me to Fuji Photo Optical (currently Fujinon), which made prototypes of dedicated endoscopes. The clinical study results of prototypes demonstrated their usefulness, and the Fujinon double-balloon electronic endoscopy system was put on the market in November 2003 [2, 3]. Engineers at Fujinon made a great contribution to commercializing this endoscopy system. I must especially express my gratitude to Shuichi Yamataka, director of the Medical Equipment Department of Fujinon, and Tetsuo Udagawa, president of Fujinon Toshiba ES Systems.

The development of the double-balloon endoscope paralleled that of the capsule endoscope. Many people expressed concern that practical application of capsule endoscopes in the near future would make the new method of enteroscope insertion obsolete. I insisted, however, that the widespread use of capsule endoscopes would not eliminate but increase the need for enteroscopes that allowed access to the entire area of the small intestine. I believed that capsule endoscopes that could reveal abnormalities would increase the need for a thorough examination by enteroscopy. My belief is now being proven [4].

The widespread use of double-balloon endoscopes and capsule endoscopes will increase interest in intestinal diseases and the need for enteroscopy. I hope this book helps popularize the technique for safe and appropriate insertion of the double-balloon endoscope.

References

1. Yamamoto H, Sekine Y, Sato Y, et al (2001) Total enteroscopy with a non-surgical steerable double-balloon method. Gastrointest Endosc 53:216–220
2. Yamamoto H, Yano T, Kita H, et al (2003) New system of double-balloon enteroscopy for diagnosis and treatment of small intestinal disorders. Gastroenterology 125:1556
3. Yamamoto H, Sugano K (2003) A new method of enteroscopy: the double-balloon method. Can J Gastroenterol 17:273–274
4. Yamamoto H, Kita H, Sunada K, et al (2004) Clinical outcomes of double-balloon endoscopy for the diagnosis and treatment of small intestinal diseases. Clin Gastroenterol Hepatol 2:1010–1016

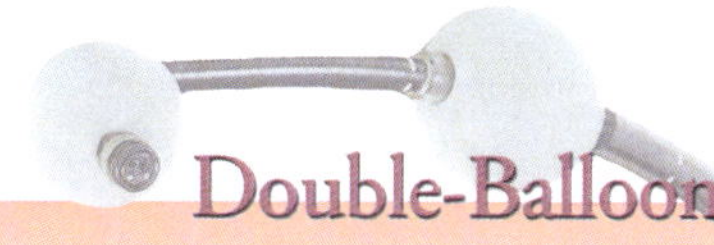

2 Equipment

2.1 Configuration

The double-balloon endoscopy system (Fig. 2.1) consists of a dedicated endoscope that can have a balloon mounted at its tip, a balloon attached to the endoscope, a balloon attached to the overtube, and a balloon pump controller to inflate and deflate the balloons (Fig. 2.2).

2.2 Devices

This subsection describes the characteristics and principle of the double-balloon endoscope distributed by Fujinon.

2.2.1 *Scope (EN-450P5, EN-450T5)*

Table 2.1 shows the specifications of the EN-450P5 and EN-450T5 scopes. Two types of dedicated scope are available. One is a standard scope with better insertability; it has a working length of 2000 mm, outer diameter of 8.5 mm, and forceps channel diameter of 2.2 mm. The other is a treatment scope with more therapeutic capabilities; it has a working length of 2000 mm, outer diameter of 9.4 mm, and forceps channel diameter of 2.8 mm

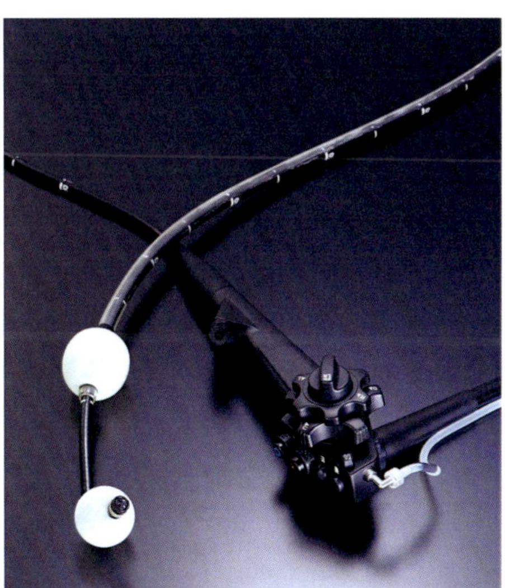

Fig. 2.1. Double-balloon endoscope

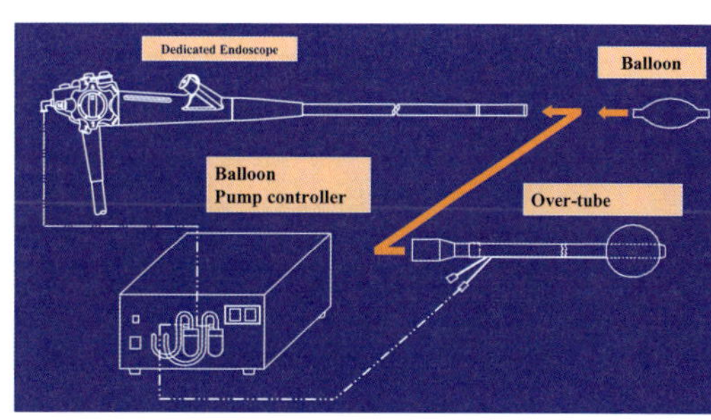

Fig. 2.2. System configuration

Table 2.1. Specifications of dedicated scopes

Variable	EN-450P5	EN-450T5
Observation range (mm)	4–100	4–100
Field of view	120°	140°
Outer diameter (mm)	8.5	9.4
Forceps channel (mm)	2.2	2.8
Working length (mm)	2000	2000

(Fig. 2.3). Each has a built-in air route to inflate and deflate the balloon attached to the tip (Fig. 2.4).

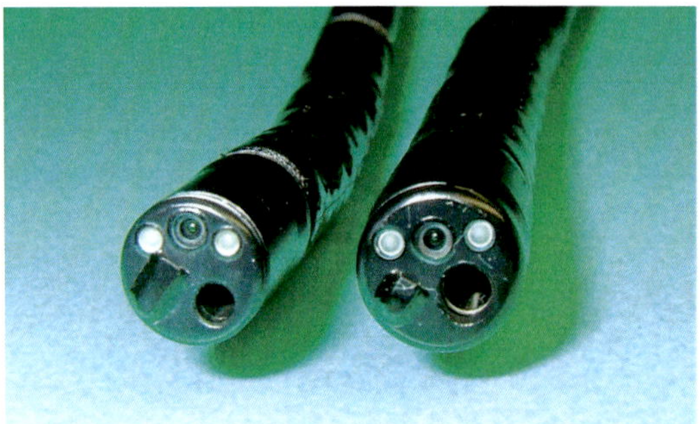

Fig. 2.3. Comparison of EN-450P5 and EN-450T5

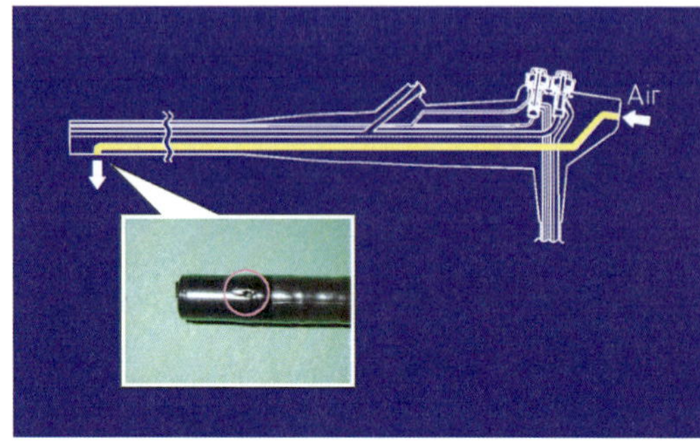

Fig. 2.4. Air route built into the scope

2.2.2 Overtube (TS-12140, TS-13140)

Two types of overtube are available. One is the TS-12140 (outer diameter 12.2 mm, length 1450 mm) for use with the EN-450P5, and the other is the TS-13140 (outer diameter 13.2 mm, length 1450 mm) for use with the EN-450T5. Both are flexible tubes. A latex balloon is mounted on the distal end of the overtube. Wetting the inner and outer surfaces of the overtube dramatically improves lubricity, which allows smooth insertion of a scope by reducing friction between the overtube and the scope and the overtube and the intestine.

As shown in Fig. 2.5, the overtube has two connection ports. The white one is connected to the balloon at the tip of the overtube through a built-in route used to inflate and deflate the balloon at the tip using a balloon pump controller, as described later. A syringe is connected to the blue connection port to inject water into the overtube, which ensures lubricity. In addition, a metal ring is embedded at the far end of the overtube with which the position of the balloon can be identified fluoroscopically.

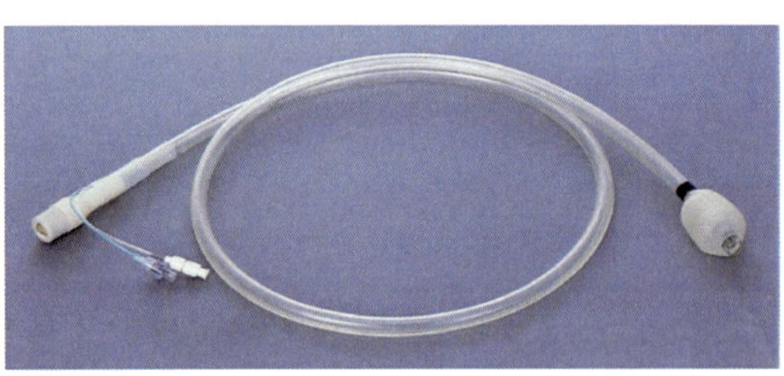

Fig. 2.5. Overtube

2.2.3 Scope Balloon (BS-1)

After the scope is passed through the overtube, a dedicated balloon (BS-1) is attached to the distal end of the scope. The balloon is made of latex and has a thickness of approximately 0.1 mm; it is designed to hold the intestine securely at the lowest possible pressure. A specifically designed device (jig) is used to attach a balloon at the distal end of the scope, and both ends of the balloon are secured with fixing rubbers. This makes the balloon ready to be inflated and deflated with a balloon pump controller that supplies and withdraws air, as shown in Fig. 2.6. Attachment procedures are detailed in Chapter 7, and illustrated in the attached DVD (digital videodisc). As needed, an ancillary dedicated hood may be attached to the distal end of the scope. Figure 2.7 shows the devices ready for use.

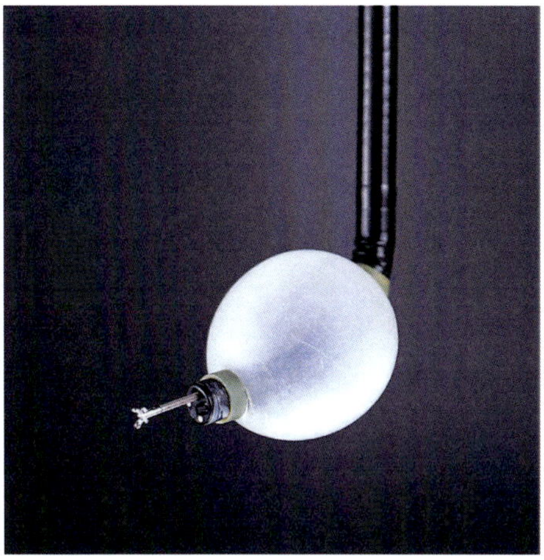

Fig. 2.6. Balloon at the scope tip

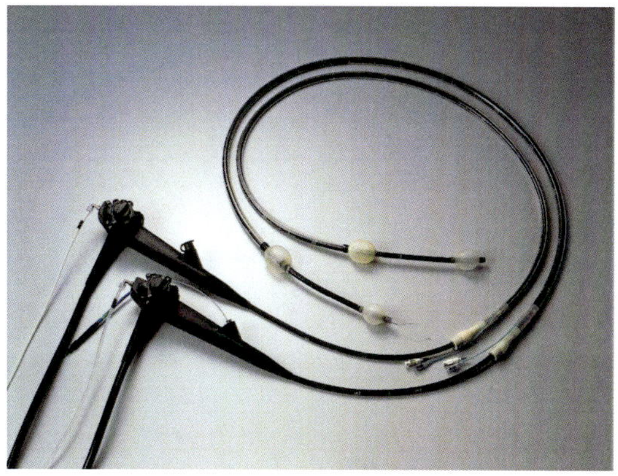

Fig. 2.7. Configuration of the scope, overtube, and balloon

2.2.4 *Balloon Pump Controller (PB-20)*

The balloon pump controller (Fig. 2.8) controls the air in the balloons on the scope and the overtube by either supplying or withdrawing air. The controller has two tubes. A transparent tube for the scope is connected to the connector on the top of the scope control head, and a white tube for the overtube is connected to the white connection port of the overtube. Air can be supplied by pushing two green buttons, one for the scope balloon and the other for the overtube balloon, on the remote switch box (inflation, LED lights up); or it can be withdrawn (deflation, LED lights off). The white buttons below the green buttons function as a pause switch to stop the air supply or withdrawal temporarily. A digital pressure monitor is on the front of the pump for monitoring balloon pressure. The balloon pressure is maintained constant at approximately 5.6 kPa (42 mm Hg) by a pressure sensing and feedback mechanism. The "level" is the minimum pressure required to anchor the intestine; a balloon inflated at such a low pressure is unlikely to cause pain or discomfort to patients.

To ensure safety, the controller is designed to activate an alarm when peristaltic movement or back-and-forth manipulation of the scope elevates the balloon pressure above a set

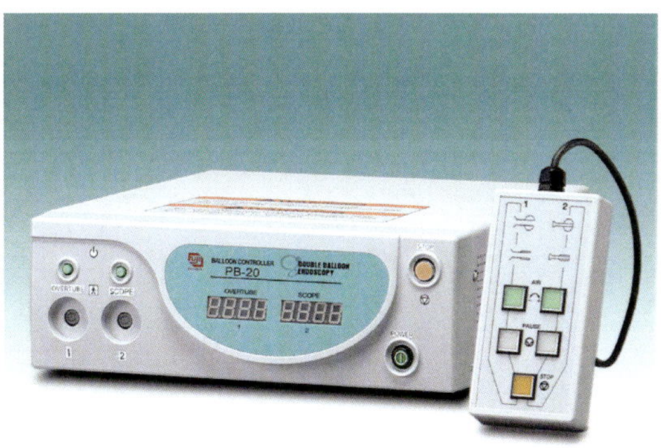

Fig. 2.8. Balloon pump controller

pressure of 8.2 kPa for 5 s or longer. The controller is also designed to sense balloon damage and air leakage from the connection, whereupon it activates an alarm. It is equipped with a filter to prevent inflow of body fluids in case of balloon damage, and due consideration is given to safety during use.

3 Indications, Contraindications, and Preoperative Examination

3.1 Indications and Contraindications

3.1.1 Indications

Double-balloon endoscopy is indicated for enteroscopy in patients who have a suspected intestinal disease and require a thorough examination to determine the treatment strategy. It is also indicated in patients who have had a confirmed diagnosis of intestinal disease and in whom endoscopic treatment is required and feasible. In addition to problems of the small intestine, double-balloon endoscopy is also indicated for examination of the entire gastrointestinal tract, which is not accessible by conventional endoscopy. The specific indications are as follows.

1. *Examination following capsule endoscopy*
   - Diagnostic endoscopy including histological examination is done for a thorough examination of suspected lesions found by capsule endoscopy.
2. *Bleeding*
   - Gastrointestinal bleeding of unknown cause ("obscure" gastrointestinal bleeding): Double-balloon endoscopy is indicated in patients with a suspected bleeding source in the small intestine that has not been identified by conventional upper gastrointestinal endoscopy or colonoscopy. Possible sites of "obscure" gastrointestinal bleeding are preferably examined carefully by skilled endoscopists because such bleeding has been reported to be attributable to lesions located within the reach of a conventional upper gastrointestinal endoscope or colonoscope in 20% of patients. If applicable, gastrointestinal bleeding scintigraphy or capsule endoscopy may be useful before undertaking double-balloon endoscopy.
   - Overt small-intestinal bleeding: Double-balloon endoscopy is indicated in patients with overt bleeding in whom bleeding sources are not identified by upper gastrointestinal endoscopy or colonoscopy. Gastrointestinal bleeding scintigraphy is preferably performed in advance to estimate the location of the bleeding site. Whether the oral or anal route is preferable is determined before enteroscopy for efficient examination on the basis of potential bleeding sites estimated by gastrointestinal bleeding scintigraphy. Where it is difficult to estimate the location of bleeding sites, one strategy is to examine most of the intestine through the anus and the remainder through the mouth because the transanal approach usually causes less discomfort (total enteroscopy is performed by using the combination). By contrast, it is often useful to select a transoral approach as a first procedure in patients with active ongoing bleeding. It is easier to identify bleeding points with the transoral approach in cases of ongoing bleeding because blood flows anally from the bleeding point in the small intestine. For hemostasis, injection and high-frequency cauterization can be performed with the EN-

450P5 enteroscope. High-frequency cauterization can be performed with the tip of a snare in the argon plasma coagulation (APC) mode (spray mode) or a hemostatic forceps in the soft coagulation mode to treat tumor bleeding, as well as hemostasis with a coagulator to treat angiectasia (angiodysplasia). The treatment-type EN-450T5 has a forceps channel with a diameter of 2.8 mm, which allows almost all endoscopic hemostasis procedures, including clips, APC probes, and other accessories. Because of the thin intestinal wall and high risk of perforation, it is deemed safe and effective to perform high-frequency cauterization after injection.

- Postoperative disorders of the gastrointestinal tract: Double-balloon endoscopy is indicated in patients with protein loss and bleeding who are suspected of having blind loop syndrome. Abdominal computed tomography, gastrointestinal bleeding scintigraphy, or albumin scintigraphy should also be performed if indicated. A capsule endoscope usually cannot access the blind loop. Multiple ulcers may occur in the afferent loop or the blind loop after gastrointestinal surgery, such as Roux-en-Y anastomosis and intestinal bypass surgery.

3. *Endoscopic diagnosis and treatment of stenosis*
   - Stenosis is a contraindication to capsule endoscopy but a good indication for double-balloon endoscopy.
   - An endoscopic or pathological diagnosis in patients with stenosis or other abnormalities revealed by small bowel series indicates the need for double-balloon endoscopy.
   - Balloon dilatation for the treatment of benign stenosis associated with Crohn's disease or other inflammatory disorders. A through-the-scope (TTS) balloon dilator is available with the EN-450T5 enteroscope.
   - Metallic stenting for palliative treatment of malignant stenosis of the small intestine. A commercially available metallic stent delivery system may require modification to ensure an adequate working length.
4. *Tumors and masses*
   - Endoscopic or pathological diagnosis of tumors or masses suspected by contrast-enhanced studies, abdominal computed tomography, or other modalities.
   - Preoperative marking in patients who are scheduled to undergo surgical resection (tattooing).
   - Hemostasis for bleeding from tumors, such as gastrointestinal stromal tumors (GISTs) or malignant lymphomas.
   - Endoscopic mucosal resection (EMR) for an intraepithelial neoplasm of the small intestine. A short overtube may be used with a double-balloon endoscope, which is replaced with another endoscope with a large channel diameter by leaving the overtube in place, thereby allowing the use of conventional therapeutic devices, although the indication is restricted by the location of lesions. The EN-450T5 allows clipping and safe EMR without changing endoscopes.
   - Polypectomy of polyps of the small intestine.
5. *Pancreatic and biliary diseases*
   - Endoscopic retrograde cholangiopancreatography (ERCP) after a Billroth II or Roux-en-Y operation.
   - Stenting or other endoscopic biliary treatment in patients with bile duct stones or tumors that are not easily accessible to a conventional endoscope because of previous intestinal reconstruction, such as a Roux-en-Y anastomosis.
6. *Crohn's disease*
   - Balloon dilatation for stenosis of the small intestine.
   - Endoscopic and histological diagnosis of Crohn's disease involving the small intestine and subsequent follow-up (contrast-enhanced studies may be sufficient). With respect to endoscopic diagnosis, capsule endoscopy may be performed as a screening method

in individuals with suspected Crohn's disease, although there is a possibility of capsule retention in the case of stenosis.

7. *Removal of a foreign body from the small intestine*
   - Removal of a foreign body from the small intestine with a basket forceps or three-pronged forceps.
   - Retrieval of a retained capsule endoscope.
   - Removal of parasites.
8. *Identification of the cause of intestinal obstruction*
   - After decompression with a long decompression tube, an overtube is inserted using a long decompression tube as a guide. After the overtube is fixed with the balloon at the tip, a long decompression tube is removed and an enteroscope is inserted. This procedure allows advancement of the enteroscope to the stenotic site within a few minutes.
   - The procedure described above allows endoscopic observation and tissue sampling through the mouth if a long decompression tube is advanced close to the lesion in patients with intestinal obstruction in whom the diagnosis is difficult to make with a colonoscope.
9. *Intussusception*
   - The anal approach allows endoscopic and histological diagnosis of the lesion inducing the intussusception. The intussuscepted intestine may be reduced or corrected by a combination of the following procedures: anchoring the intestine in place with a balloon, exerting manual pressure, and injecting contrast medium. The possibility of intestinal ischemia should be excluded before attempting the correction.
10. *Difficult colonoscopy*
    - Double-balloon endoscopy is applicable in patients who have undergone a difficult colonoscopy especially due to adhesions that precluded straightening the sigmoid or transverse colon. Dolichocolon without adhesions or other conditions for which total colonoscopy is technically difficult is also a good indication. Supporting the sagged intestinal tract with the balloon-attached overtube allows deep insertion of the endoscope while preventing it from further stretching the intestine.

3.1.2 *Contraindications*

Contraindications to the use of the double-balloon endoscope are essentially similar to those for the use of conventional upper gastrointestinal endoscopes and colonoscopes. Endoscopy is indicated only if the potential benefit outweighs the potential risk in patients in poor general condition, those with a risk of gastrointestinal perforation, or patients with significant respiratory or cardiovascular disease. Endoscopy should not be performed in individuals who refuse to undergo the procedure after giving fully informed consent. Meticulous care should be exercised when the endoscope is advanced beyond lesions such as strictures, deep ulcers, or large tumors, although these conditions are not absolute contraindications. It should be noted that there is still a possibility that balloon inflation as well as stretching and shortening operations during endoscopy might result in perforation of fragile, affected regions of the intestine, although the pressure of the balloon is controlled at less than 45 mm Hg during the whole procedure. Deeper insertion of the endoscope should not be forced, especially in these cases.

3.2 Preoperative Examination

Preoperative interviews and examinations should include the following: a review of stool color (by interview or rectal examination); body weight (to determine the sedatives' doses);

medical history, such as past history (previous abdominal surgery, trauma, accident); the presence or absence of previous anesthesia and its related complications; previous drug allergies; the presence or absence of contraindications to anticholinergic agents, such as ischemic heart disease, glaucoma, prostatic hypertrophy; review of oral medications [use of anticoagulants or nonsteroidal antiinflammatory drugs (NSAIDs)]; blood coagulation tests; thoracic and abdominal radiography; and electrocardiography.

It is particularly important to interview patients regarding their use of NSAIDs. Many of the patients taking NSAIDs are older individuals who are unaware of the name and action of medications. These drugs have often been prescribed at multiple medical institutions, and some patients take their medications without knowing that they are "painkillers." Their medications should therefore be reviewed by contacting the medical institutions at which the patients have undergone outpatient treatment. In patients with current or previous use of NSAIDs, NSAID-induced enterocolitis should be taken into consideration at the examination. Etodolac, meloxicam, and other agents with high selectivity for cyclooxygenase-2 are preferentially prescribed for orthopedic disorders, and their unlimited use may lead to iron deficiency anemia or hypoproteinemia "unknown cause". Recently developed capsule endoscopy has shown that patients taking NSAIDs are more likely to have lesions in the small intestine compared with a control group; and it is preferable that endoscopists and gastroenterologists enlighten other physicians on possible NSAID-induced small-intestinal disorders. Patients with intestinal stenosis should be interviewed about previous abdominal contusions associated with traffic accidents or falls, which may have caused mesenteric injury and subsequent ischemic stenosis. The type of abdominal surgery and the procedure should be reviewed, particularly when the surgery involves the intestine. Blind loop syndrome should be taken into consideration in patients with previous intestinal surgery. Thus, the medical interview often helps identify lesions in the small intestine.

Conventional modalities that are potentially useful for diagnosis should also be considered, depending on the case. Such modalities include upper gastrointestinal endoscopy, colonoscopy, contrast-enhanced studies of the gastrointestinal tract (double-contrast examination of the small intestine), abdominal computed tomography (plain and contrast-enhanced), abdominal magnetic resonance imaging (MRI), α_1-antitrypsin test of feces, nuclear medicine examinations (including gastrointestinal bleeding scintigraphy, albumin scintigraphy, Meckel's scintigraphy, gallium scintigraphy, positron emission tomography), and abdominal angiography.

Review of previous films is also important. Particularly, a diagnosis using double-contrast examination of the small intestine is difficult, and abnormalities may be overlooked. To prevent an oversight, the diagnosis is preferably made by multiple physicians.

To identify a source of bleeding, ^{99m}Tc-labeled red blood cell scintigraphy can reveal persistent bleeding of as little as 0.1 ml/min, and abdominal angiography can detect as little as 0.5 ml/min. Although double-balloon endoscopy is relatively minimally invasive, a thorough examination of the entire small intestine requires considerable effort, and thus information on a rough estimation about the location of the abnormality helps improve the accuracy of the examination. Therefore, in a patient with gastrointestinal bleeding, scintigraphy, capsule endoscopy, or other procedures should be considered before double-balloon endoscopy is undertaken.

Effective examinations can be performed by narrowing the choice of possible locations of lesions and by determining the approach route based on the results of these examinations. When no factors are available to determine whether the oral or anal approach is better, the anal approach should be selected because the patient is less likely to experience discomfort. An enteroscope is inserted through the anus, and tattooing is performed at the deepest site reached; the subsequent examination may be done through the mouth.

Reference

1. The Japan Gastroenterological Endoscopy Society (2002) Guidelines for gastroenterological endoscopy, 2nd edn. Igaku-Shoin, Tokyo

4 Informed Consent

Informed consent means understanding and consenting to a procedure on the basis of an adequate explanation. It is a process by which health care providers give the patient easy-to-understand information about the nature and necessity of the examination and treatment, allow the patient to choose among alternatives, and obtain consent from the patient to perform the procedure. In the field of gastrointestinal endoscopy, it is now common practice to obtain informed consent and maintain written consent for relatively invasive operations, including endoscopic retrograde cholangiopancreatography, polypectomy, and endoscopic mucosal resection. Moreover, an increasing number of institutions also obtain written consent for routine upper or lower endoscopy. An increase in the number of endoscopic examinations is associated with more complications during the examination and treatment, greater public interest, and an increase in medical lawsuits. The role of informed consent should be well understood in the context of these circumstances.

4.1 Informed Consent Procedures

Informed consent procedures may include an oral explanation and documentation on the patient's chart. It is advisable to prepare written information about the examination in advance to provide patients with easy-to-understand information in busy clinical settings. Information may be provided with the use of illustrated written information, videotapes of the examination, or presentation software and a computer monitor. Our institution uses written information that simply illustrates the principle of endoscope insertion into the distal small intestine (Fig. 4.1).

4.2 Details of Informed Consent

The primary information provided during informed consent procedures should include the objectives, procedures, complications, and the patient's human rights.

4.2.1 *Objective*

The reason the examination is to be performed should be clearly presented. It is necessary to describe the advantages of double-balloon endoscopy over other modalities. Double-balloon endoscopy allows relatively easy access to lesions located deep in the small intestine, which is not accessible with the conventional push method. It also allows treatment of emergencies, such as small-intestinal bleeding, in a timely manner. It enables not only observation but also biopsy and treatment of lesions. These potential advantages should be explained in association with patients' current conditions.

• Information on insertion of an enteroscope with two balloons (double-balloon enteroscopy)

1. *Objective.*
Double-balloon enteroscopy is an examination in which an endoscope is inserted through the mouth or the anus into the small intestine for the diagnosis of diseases in the small intestine. The examination is performed to diagnose bleeding, inflammation (enterocolitis), tumors, and narrowing of the small intestine. The examination may be accompanied by treatment to stop bleeding or to dilate a narrowing. This procedure may be performed as colonoscopy in patients in whom a conventional colonoscope failed to advance far enough.

2. *Procedures.*
The endoscope (at right) used has a structure similar to that of conventional gastroscopes and colonoscopes, but it is longer than gastroscopes and colonoscopes because of the distance of the small intestine from the mouth and the anus. We have developed a method for inserting an endoscope with two balloons, a type of "measuring worm," to insert the endoscope more safely and reliably into the entire small intestine. We have performed the procedure in many patients. This endoscopic system consists of an endoscope with a balloon at its tip and a balloon-attached overtube. The endoscope advances into the small intestine like a "measuring worm" while the distance between the balloon of the endoscope and that of the covering overtube is increased and decreased (see an attached information sheet for specific insertion procedures). Sedative and pain-killing medications are used to reduce pain during the examination, which takes about 1–2 h.

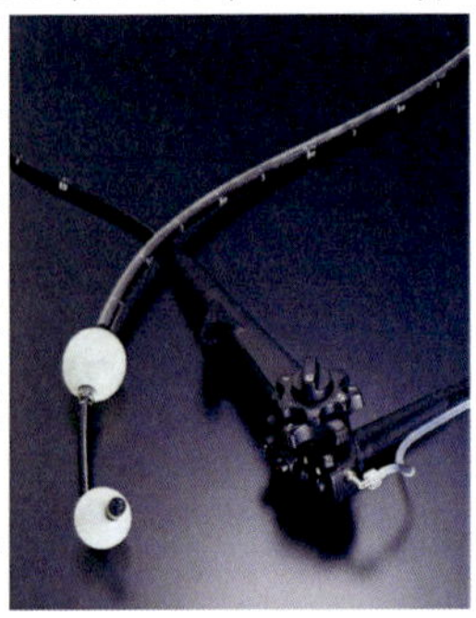

Double-balloon endoscope is on the *right*

a

3. *Complications.*
Complications of conventional endoscopy may occur, such as pain, nausea, vomiting, and bleeding. In particular, patients with prior abdominal surgery, including gynecologic surgery, may experience pain during endoscopy. Rarely, gastrointestinal perforation (a hole in the gastrointestinal tract) may require emergency surgery. Extremely rarely, the use of sedatives may be associated with complications of aspiration (inhalation of saliva or vomit into the lungs) and resultant aspiration pneumonia, respiratory arrest, and cardiac arrest (in the event of these complications, emergency measures are available).
Between September 25, 2000 and January 31, 2004 we performed 178 double-balloon endoscopic examinations on 123 patients, none of whom experienced respiratory or cardiac arrest during the examination.

4. *Patients may refuse to undergo the examination or treatment without penalty.*
Patients have the choice of whether to undergo this examination. Patients refusing the examination are allowed to receive other treatments without penalty at our hospital.

5. *Patients consenting to the examination or treatment are free to withdraw their consent at any time.*

6. *Other considerations required to protect patients' rights.*
This treatment must be voluntary, and patients' willingness is the first priority in regard to performing the treatment. Please feel free to ask any questions about the procedures.

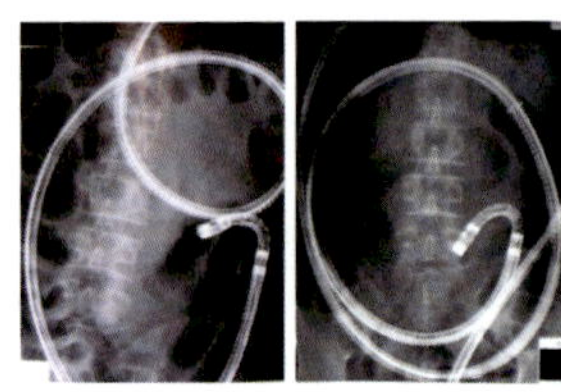

Left Radiograph showing an enteroscope inserted through the mouth
Right Radiograph showing an enteroscope inserted through the anus

b

• Informed consent form for double-balloon endoscopy

☐Enteroscopy ☐Colonoscopy

I have been fully informed by Dr. ______ and understand the objective, procedures, expected benefits, and complications of double-balloon endoscopy as well as the availability, benefits, and complications of other procedures. I voluntarily consent to undergo this examination. I also understand that I may withdraw my consent at any time without penalty.

Date: ____________

Patient: ____________________ (seal)

Address: ____________________

____

Relative (relationship): ________ (seal)

Address: ____________________

____

Jichi Medical University, Department of Gastroenterology

c

• Insertion of the double-balloon enteroscope through the mouth

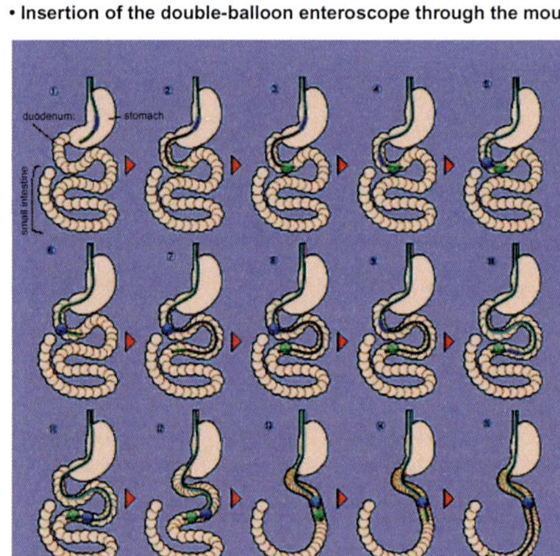

1. The endoscope is inserted into the stomach.
2. The endoscope tip is inserted into the duodenum. These procedures are similar to those for the gastroscope.
3. The balloon (*green*) at the endoscope tip inserted into the duodenum is inflated to anchor the intestine from the inside.
4. Along the endoscope, the overtube tip is advanced close to the endoscope tip.
5. The overtube balloon (*blue*) is inflated.
6. The balloon (*green*) at the endoscope tip is deflated.
7. The endoscope is moved more deeply. The overtube balloon anchoring the intestinal tract from inside allows smooth insertion of the endoscope to a deeper point.

d

Fig. 4.1a–g. Information to be given to patients to obtain informed consent for double-balloon endoscopy (Jichi Medical University)

8. After the endoscope is advanced more deeply, the endoscope balloon (*green*) is inflated again to anchor the intestinal tract from the inside.
9. The overtube balloon (*blue*) is deflated.
10. Along the endoscope, the overtube tip is again advanced close to the endoscope tip.
11. The overtube balloon (*blue*) is inflated.
12, 13. Both balloons are inflated to anchor the intestinal tract from the inside, and the entire endoscope is pulled back to shorten the small intestine.
14, 15. The balloon (*green*) at the endoscope tip is again deflated, and the endoscope is inserted more deeply.
16. Steps 8–15 are then repeated to insert the endoscope farther into the small intestine.

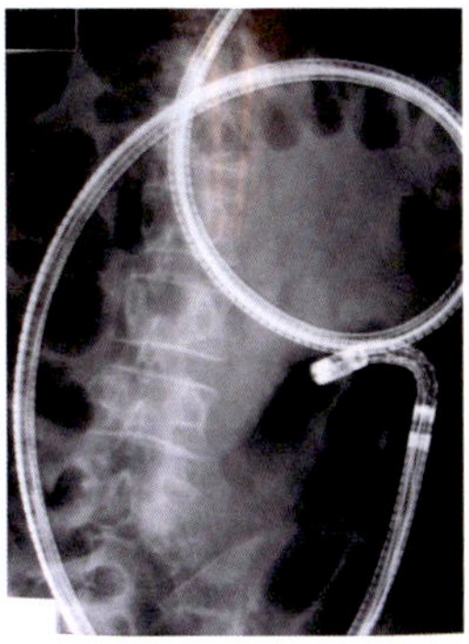

Radiograph showing an endoscope inserted through the mouth into the middle of the small intestine for a total distance of 7–8 m

e

• Insertion of the double-balloon enteroscope or colonoscope through the anus

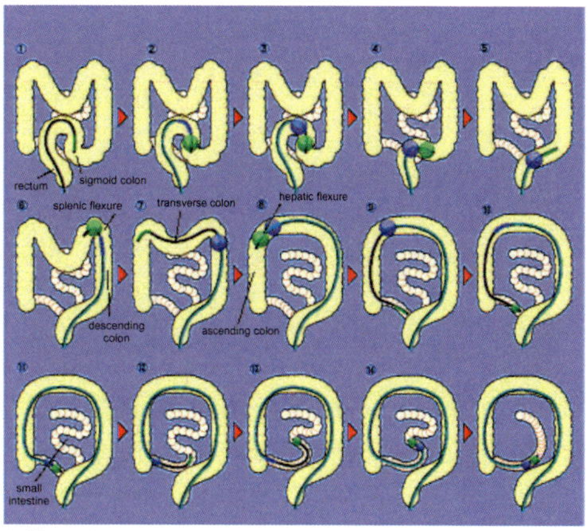

1. The endoscope is inserted into the rectum or the sigmoid colon. This procedure is similar to that for conventional colonoscopy.
2. The balloon (*green*) at the endoscope tip is inflated to anchor the intestine from the inside.
3. With the endoscope as a guide, the overtube tip is advanced close to the endoscope tip, and the overtube balloon (*blue*) is also inflated.
4. Both the endoscope and the overtube are pulled back to reduce bends and straighten the rectum and sigmoid colon.
5. The balloon (*green*) at the endoscope tip is deflated, and the endoscope tip is moved more deeply.
6. The balloon (*green*) at the endoscope tip is inflated to secure the endoscope tip in the splenic flexure. The overtube balloon is deflated, and the overtube alone is advanced along the endoscope until it reaches the endoscope tip.

f

7. The overtube balloon (*blue*) is inflated, the balloon (*green*) at the endoscope tip is deflated, and the endoscope tip is moved more deeply. The overtube balloon (*blue*) anchoring the intestinal tract from the inside allows smooth insertion of the endoscope farther into the small intestine.
8. When the endoscope tip reaches the hepatic flexure, the balloon (*green*) at the endoscope tip is inflated. The overtube balloon (*blue*) is deflated, the overtube is again advanced to the endoscope tip, and the balloon (*blue*) is reinflated. With both balloons inflated, the endoscope and the overtube are pulled back simultaneously to reduce the bends and loops of the transverse colon and to straighten it.
9. The balloon (*green*) at the endoscope tip is deflated, and the endoscope tip is advanced farther into the small intestine.
10. The balloon (*green*) at the endoscope tip is inflated to secure the endoscope tip.
11. After the balloon (*blue*) at the overtube tip is deflated, the overtube tip is again advanced close to the endoscope tip with the endoscope as a guide, and the balloon (*blue*) at the overtube tip is reinflated.
12. The balloon (*green*) at the endoscope tip is deflated, and the endoscope tip is inserted more deeply into the small intestine.
13. The balloon (*green*) at the endoscope tip is inflated to anchor the intestinal tract.
14. After the balloon (*blue*) at the overtube tip is deflated, the overtube tip is again advanced close to the endoscope tip with the endoscope as a guide, and the balloon at the overtube tip is reinflated.
15. Both balloons are inflated to anchor the intestinal tract from the inside, and the entire endoscope is pulled back to shorten the small intestine.
16. Steps 12–15 are repeated to insert the endoscope more deeply.

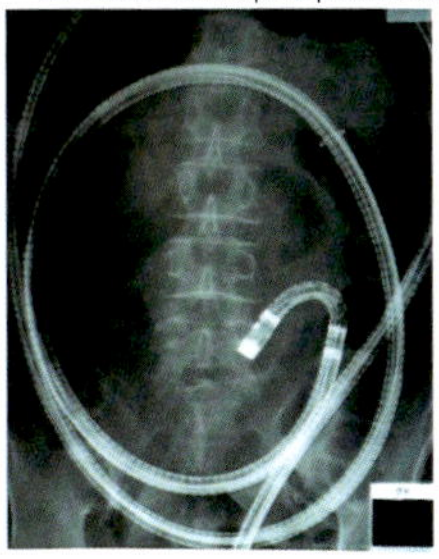

Radiograph showing an endoscope inserted through the anus into the middle of the small intestine for a total distance of 7–8 m

g

4.2.2 *Procedures*

First, the principle of insertion should be described in plain language. Illustrations are preferable for showing the structure of the endoscope and the anatomy. It is desirable that patients understand how the double-balloon endoscope is inserted into the deep small intestine. Next, actual examination procedures are described step by step. Technical terms are avoided to ensure that patients get the whole picture of the examination procedure, including the use of sedatives, positioning for the examination, use of fluoroscopy, the time required for the examination, and safety monitoring procedures.

4.2.3 *Complications*

There is an increasing demand for disclosure of specific information about complications. *Guidelines for Gastroenterological Endoscopy*, developed by the Japanese Society of Gastroenterology [1], indicate that physicians should consider it essential to provide information about complications, including their nature and frequency, the possible need for surgery, and the associated mortality. Double-balloon endoscopy is a newly developed procedure, and evaluation of its safety must await the accrual of patients undergoing the procedure. The lack of nationwide statistics on complications makes it difficult to describe complications on the basis of specific figures. Patients should be well informed of foreseeable complications, including bleeding, gastrointestinal perforation, and those related to such medications as anesthetics for the throat and sedatives, as well as specific emergency treatments.

4.2.4 *Patients' Human Rights*

It should be stipulated that patients who do not consent to undergo the examination still have a right to alternative examinations or treatments without penalty, and due consideration must be given to the patients' human rights. Patients must be allowed to have the choice, and the examination must be voluntary.

4.3 Details of Written Consent

Written consent is required that demonstrates the patient's full understanding of the nature of the examination and his or her consent. Written consent forms typically come with written information that describes the objectives, procedures, and complications. Entries on the form should include the date and time that information is provided and the names of the physicians and others present, the patient giving consent, and a member of his or her family. The written consent consists of two sheets of paper; one is filed in the patient's chart and the other is for the patient.

Adequate information provides patients with a sense of security, resulting in a safe examination. Informed consent represents not only the physician's accountability but also an important process by which a trustful relationship develops between the physician and the patient.

Reference

1. The Japan Gastroenterological Endoscopy Society (2002) Guidelines for gastroenterological endoscopy, 2nd edn. Igaku-Shoin, Tokyo

5 Principle of Insertion and Characteristics

Double-Balloon

5.1 Principle of Insertion of the Double-Balloon Endoscope

In general, the most important factor when inserting an endoscope is to transmit the force applied to the endoscope shaft effectively to the endoscope tip. When the endoscope bends intricately or forms a loop, the force applied to the endoscope shaft is not transmitted to the endoscope tip, and thus the endoscope tip does not advance. When an enteroscope is inserted by the push method (the most commonly used technique for enteroscope insertion), the enteroscope may bend intricately or form a loop. Attempts were made to straighten the intestine with an inflexible overtube to prevent bend and loop formation and to insert an endoscope into the distal small intestine. However, it is impossible to straighten the entire small intestine, and it is harmful to straighten the intestine forcibly.

In fact, insertion is difficult not because of the bends and loops of an endoscope but because of stretching that part of the intestinal tract that forms a bend or a loop. Insertion of the endoscope shaft stretches the intestine, but the force is not effectively transmitted to the endoscope tip, thereby failing to advance the tip (Fig. 5.1). Unless this problem is solved, a simple endoscope with a long working length cannot reach the deep small intestine.

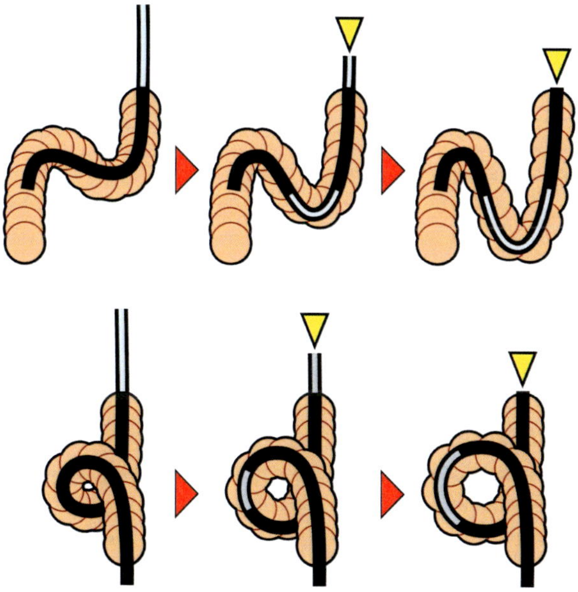

Fig. 5.1. Stretching a curved or looped intestine

This problem can be solved by avoiding stretching of the intestinal tract through which the endoscope tip has passed. Double-balloon endoscopy uses a flexible overtube with a balloon at its tip to prevent the stretching. The inflated balloon at the tip of the overtube anchors the intestine in place from inside and prevents the tip of the overtube from slipping. The overtube can bend flexibly but not stretch. The overtube does not stretch even in the presence of bends or loops, and neither does the intestinal tract that is being anchored by the balloon at the tip of the overtube. Consequently, insertion of the endoscope shaft does not stretch the intestine, and the force is effectively transmitted to the endoscope tip. Thus, the endoscope can be advanced into the deep portion of the small intestine, with the balloon at the tip of the overtube as a fixed support (Fig. 5.2).

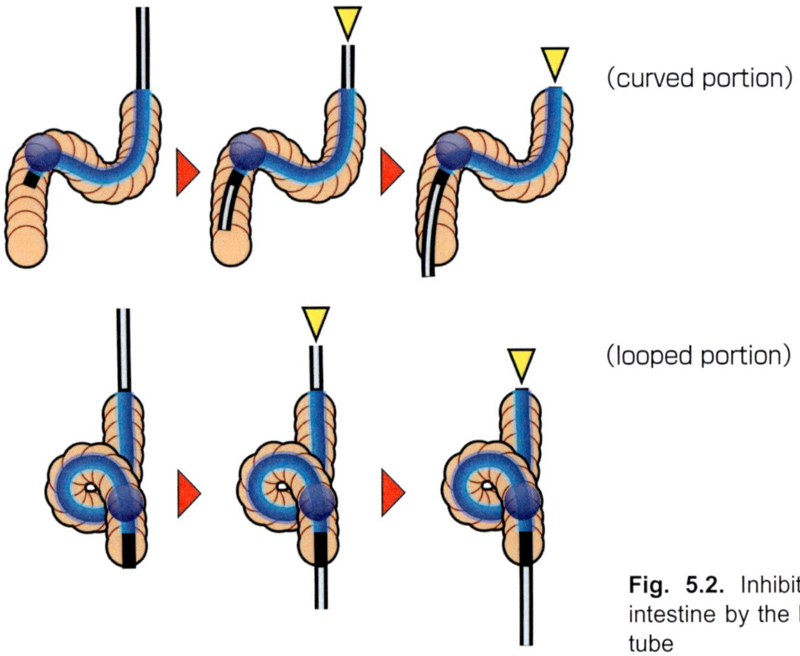

Fig. 5.2. Inhibition of stretching the intestine by the balloon-attached overtube

During double-balloon endoscopy the endoscope is advanced as deeply as possible; the balloon at the tip of the overtube is then deflated, and the overtube is slid distally onto the endoscope. During the procedure, the balloon at the endoscope tip is inflated to grip the intestine from inside, preventing the endoscope tip from slipping. After deflating the balloon at the tip of the overtube and sliding the overtube to the deep position, the balloon at the tip of the overtube is inflated, and the endoscope and the overtube are withdrawn with the two balloons inflated. Through this procedure the inserted intestinal tract is pleated over the overtube and thus shortened (Fig. 5.3). The procedures are repeated to make the best use of the endoscope's working length and shorten the intestine of a total length of 6–7 m, enabling observation of the intestine with the endoscope with a working length of 200 cm. Moreover, the shortening procedure simplifies the curved intestine ahead as well as the subsequent insertion procedure (Fig. 5.4).

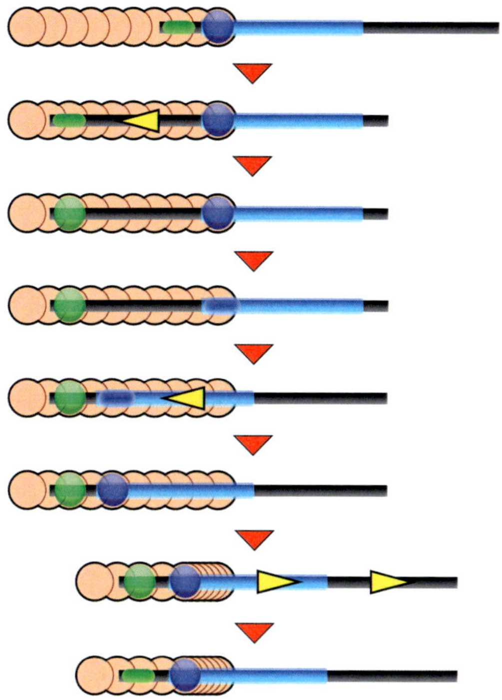

Fig. 5.3. Shortening the intestine with two balloons

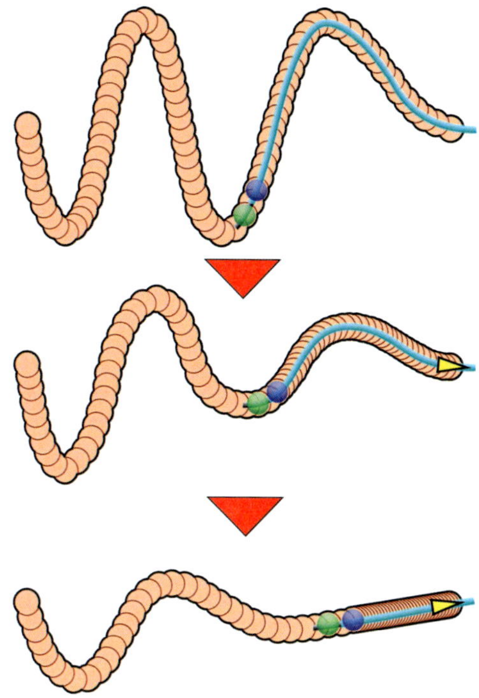

Fig. 5.4. Simplifying the shape of the intestine ahead

In short, double-balloon endoscopy takes advantage of the free mobility of the small intestine (which is not fixed in the abdominal cavity), shortens the small intestine, and simplifies the shape of the small intestine ahead. The endoscope is inserted deeper into the small intestine while the fixed support established by the balloon at the tip of the overtube is moved step by step.

5.2 Characteristics of the Double-Balloon Endoscope

Although a conventional endoscope with a long working length generates concern about maneuverability, the tip of the double-balloon endoscope can be manipulated with the help of a fixed point supported by the balloon at the tip of the overtube. This enables free back-and-forth observation without sacrifice of maneuverability no matter how deeply the endoscope is inserted. Moreover, this method allows insertion from both the mouth and the anus because insertion does not depend on peristalsis of the intestine. Observation of a surgically bypassed segment of the intestine is not possible by the ropeway method, sonde method, or even capsule endoscopy; but it is possible with the double-balloon endoscope.

The tip of the double-balloon endoscope has bending capability (up and down, left and right) and a forceps channel; and it allows directed biopsy, which cannot be performed by the ropeway method or the sonde method. Endoscopic treatment can be performed with a therapeutic device. A therapeutic device with a large diameter may be used without being restricted by the forceps channel diameter after removal of the endoscope with the overtube left in place. The use of a double-balloon endoscope allows endoscopic treatment of lesions in any portion of the small intestine.

It should be noted that this procedure dramatically reduces the patient's discomfort related to endoscopy compared with the push method. Most endoscopy-related discomfort is due to stretching the curved or looped portion of the intestine. Double-balloon endoscopy causes less discomfort due to stretching of the intestine because the method, in principle, allows insertion while inhibiting stretching of the intestine.

6 Preparation and Premedication

6.1 Preparation

6.1.1 Double-Balloon Endoscopy Through the Mouth

Double-balloon endoscopy through the mouth allows insertion of the scope to the jejunoileal junction in many cases and occasionally into the terminal ileum or even the large intestine. After about 12 h of fasting, food residue usually reaches the large intestine. We have rarely found food residue in the small intestine in patients fasting only on the day of the examination as in the case of routine upper endoscopy. Pale yellow intestinal fluids do not interfere with the insertion or the examination. When no cathartic is used and stool remains in the large intestine, however, the examination may be associated with a patient being embarrassed because of the increased abdominal pressure and a high incidence of vagal reflex activity, both of which are avoidable. In addition, some examinations require the use of a contrast agent (meglumine sodium amidotrizoate), which may increase intestinal peristalsis, stimulate defecation, and interfere with the examination. Thus, it is desirable to empty the intestinal tract, including the large intestine, with a regular laxative and a suppository or enema. Unlike the preparation for colonoscopy, it is not necessary to cleanse the mucosal surface with a bowel cleansing solution.

Example of a prescription

sodium picosulfate (regular laxative): 0.75% 10 ml p.o. on the night before the examination

sodium bicarbonate, anhydrous monobasic sodium phosphate (suppository) : 2.6g one piece on the morning of the examination

6.1.2 Double-Balloon Endoscopy Through the Anus

Double-balloon endoscopy through the anus requires emptying the large intestine because the endoscope reaches the ileum via the large intestine. The intestine should be free of large scybala, as even a small amount of residue may stick to the endoscope and move into the overtube, thereby increasing friction. As in the case of colonoscopy, cloudy intestinal fluids impair visibility and make insertion difficult. For these reasons, when performing double-balloon endoscopy through the anus, we use the bowel-cleansing solution (polyethylene glycol electrolyte solution), as in the case of colonoscopy.

Example of a prescription

sennoside: 12mg two tablets at bedtime on the day before the examination

polyethylene glycol electrolyte solution: 137.155 g one pack dissolved in 2 l of water and administered over a period of 2 h or more.

6.1.3 Postoperative Stomach

Food residue may remain in the stomach at the time of upper endoscopy in patients with a history of subtotal gastrectomy because of impaired peristalsis of the residual stomach. Fine food residue remaining in the stomach may fill the space between the overtube and the enteroscope, generate friction, and make insertion difficult. Conventional upper endoscopy should be performed in advance in patients with a history of gastrectomy to examine for reconstruction and food residue. When residue is found, a cathartic and appropriate diet should be used before enteroscopy.

6.2 Premedication

6.2.1 Sedation

In Japan, fewer institutions are using intravenous sedation to prepare for upper gastrointestinal endoscopy. By contrast, an increasing number of institutions are administering sedation to reduce the discomfort associated with insertion of a colonoscope [1].

Double-balloon endoscopy substantially reduces patient discomfort compared with conventional push enteroscopy because it allows insertion while avoiding intestinal stretching, but it is still not an entirely noninvasive procedure. The whole procedure takes 1–2 h, and insertion and shortening cause some discomfort in the abdomen or the throat. Despite adequate information before the examination, patients are more likely to experience anxiety than with conventional endoscopy because many of them have not undergone this examination.

It is the responsibility of the endoscopist to perform painless, comfortable endoscopy on patients, and it is therefore important to administer appropriate sedation. The optimal level of sedation for endoscopy is conscious sedation, which is defined as a sedative condition where the patient retains the ability to communicate verbally with the physician [1]. Conscious sedation is advantageous in that the drugs exert anxiolytic and amnesic effects, the endoscopy is performed while monitoring the patient's condition, sedatives can be added as needed, and it requires minimal monitoring [2].

6.2.2 Types of Premedication

Medications used for sedation are classified into sedatives and analgesics. Most sedatives

Table 6.1. Types of premedication

Generic name	Trade name	Dose	Reversal agent
Sedatives			
Diazepam	Cercine, Horizon	5–10 mg	Flumazenil
Midazolam	Dormicum	0.15–0.3 mg/kg	Flumazenil
Flunitrazepam	Silece, Rohypnol	0.01–0.03 mg/kg	Flumazenil
Analgesics			
Pethidine HCl	Opystan	35 mg	Naloxone HCl
Pentazocine	Sosegon, Pentagin	15 mg	Naloxone HCl
Buprenorphine	Lepetan	0.2–0.4 mg	

are benzodiazepines, with representative drugs such as diazepam, midazolam, and flunitrazepam. Analgesics include pethidine hydrochloride, pentazocine, and buprenorphine (Table 6.1).

Benzodiazepines used for sedation are characterized by their rapid onset of central nervous system effects. They can induce sedation, hypnosis, sleep, and respiratory depression, which require adequate cardiopulmonary management. A certain level of anesthesia may induce excitation (increased body movement) by disinhibition of the limbic system, so caution should be exercised. These agents are lipid-soluble and are metabolized in the liver; thus, care should be exercised in older individuals and patients with liver disease. Flumazenil is an effective reversal agent; however, it has a short half-life, and respiratory depression could recur after recovery. The analgesic pethidine hydrochloride is a narcotic drug, and its use requires specific formalities. It has a rapid onset of action at an intravenous dose of 35 mg and is frequently used during endoscopy. Adverse reactions include dizziness, nausea, vomiting, and respiratory depression; dose adjustment is important in patients with chronic respiratory disease and older individuals.

6.2.3 Dosage and Administration

Specifically, we start with intravenous administration of pethidine hydrochloride (1 ampule of Opystan, 35 mg/ampule) in combination with diazepam (half an ampule of Horizon, 10 mg/ampule) or midazolam (half an ampule of Dormicum, 10 mg/ampule); we then administer additional doses of diazepam or midazolam as needed. Doses of analgesics and sedatives are adjusted according to the patient's age, physical constitution, and condition. In most patients, adequate sedation is achieved by this method. When body movement interferes with the examination in patients with a decreased level of consciousness, addition of pethidine hydrochloride is often effective.

Pethidine hydrochloride alone is expected to exert a spasmolytic effect to some extent. When peristalsis interferes with insertion through the anus, we intravenously administer scopolamine butylbromide as needed.

6.2.4 Monitoring

Physicians should be fully aware that sedation may be associated with a variety of adverse reactions. Particular attention should be given to respiratory depression and cardiovascular depression. The patient's condition is closely monitored during the examination, but the operator tends to concentrate on the endoscopic monitor. Preferably, one physician or endoscopy technician is dedicated solely to monitoring the patient.

The American Society for Gastrointestinal Endoscopy has reported that the combination of three devices—pulse oximeter, automated sphygmomanometer, and electrocardiograph monitor—is most useful and effective for patient management [3]. Simple attachment of the sensor to the finger of the patient allows a pulse oximeter to display blood oxygen saturation and sound an alarm when hypoxia occurs; thus, it appears to be essential during sedation. When the oxygen saturation is 90% or less, the patient should be given verbal commands repeatedly. If the stimuli are insufficient, oxygen inhalation is started. During oxygen administration, however, ventilatory insufficiency may occur in the presence of satisfactory oxygen saturation, and thus supplemental oxygen should be kept at a low level. During double-balloon endoscopy, often performed to investigate the cause of gastrointestinal bleeding or anemia, the use of an electrocardiograph monitor, blood pressure monitor, and pulse oximeter is recommended in all individuals, particularly those who are older and patients with heart disease or chronic respiratory disease.

References

1. Sawatake N, Munakata A, Sakai Y (2002) Guidelines for endoscopy in older individuals. In: Guidelines for gastroenterological endoscopy, 2nd edn. Igaku-Shoin, Tokyo, pp 157–163
2. Fujinuma S, Seike M, Ohta A, et al (2003) Use of premedication and patient management in colonoscopy. Endosc Dig 11:1587–1591
3. ASGE (1995) Technology assessment status evaluation: monitoring equipment for endoscopy. Gastrointest Endosc 42:615–617

7 Preparation of Devices

Unlike the conventional endoscopy system, the double-balloon endoscopy system consists of an endoscope, light source, overtube with balloon attached, balloon at the endoscope tip, and balloon pump controller. Although many think that checking/preparing the double-balloon endoscope requires substantial time and effort because of its complexity, the procedures are not as complicated as expected. A person familiar with the procedures can complete the checking and preparation in 10 min or so. This chapter details our routine preparation procedures for the double-balloon endoscope and related considerations.

7.1 Preparation

1. Connect a 20-ml syringe to the endoscope tube connector and flush the air route several times with air to remove any water that might cause a blockage (Fig. 7.1).

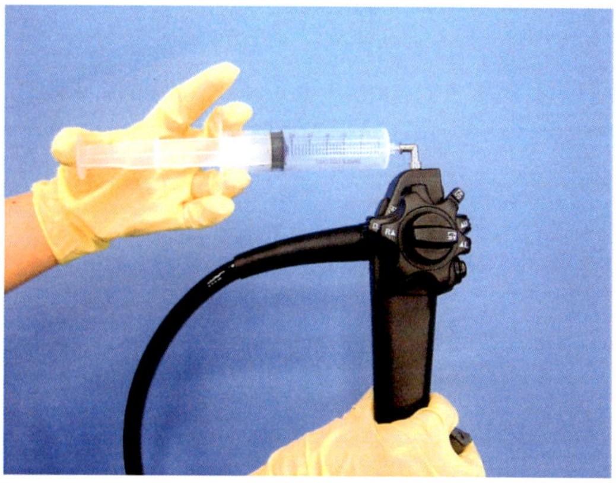

Fig. 7.1. Flush the air route with air

2. Attach a backflow check valve made of rubber (ST-03B) to the proximal end of the overtube. Adjust the length of the rubber protruding proximally to ensure that the rubber does not become entangled between the overtube and the endoscope, thereby generating resistance. Secure the rubber with surgical tape (Fig. 7.2).

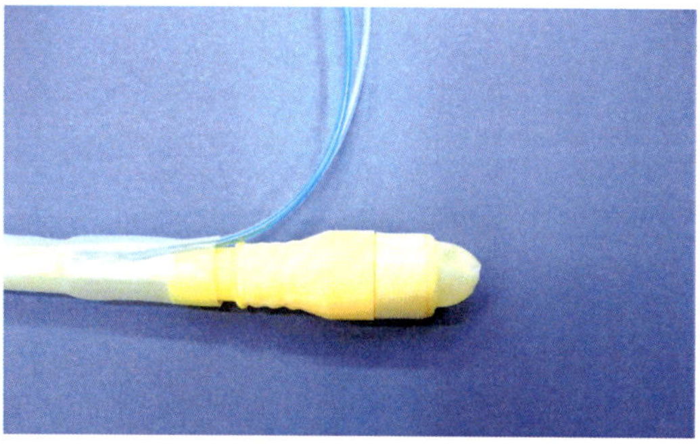

Fig. 7.2. Attach a backflow check valve made of rubber to the proximal end of the overtube

3. Connect the balloon pump controller to the overtube and the endoscope with dedicated tubes (Fig. 7.3).

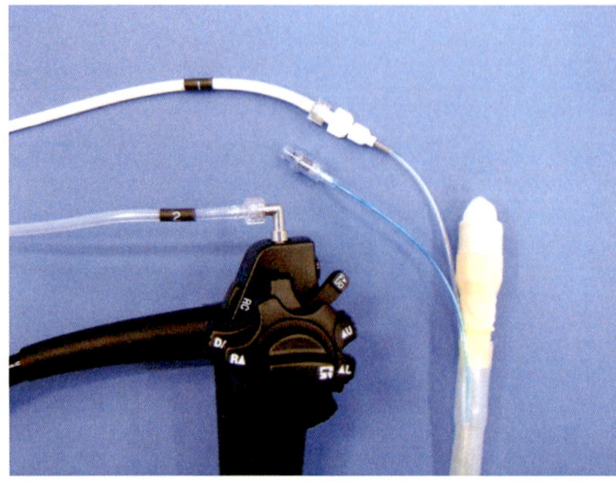

Fig. 7.3. Connect the balloon pump controller to the overtube and the endoscope with tubes

4. Turn on the power of the balloon pump controller. Press and light up the scope selector switch (2) on the remote switch box (Fig. 7.4a). Immerse the endoscope tip in a glass of water to confirm that air bubbles come out the tip (Fig. 7.4b). After confirmation, take the endoscope tip out of the water, wipe the water off the tip, and then press the scope's pause switch (4) on the remote switch box.

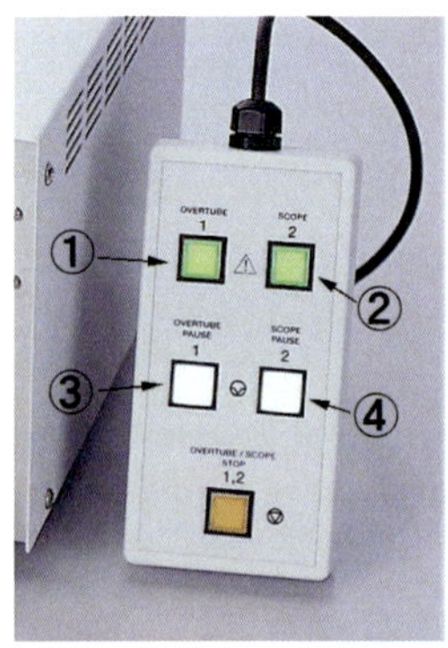

Fig. 7.4a. Remote switches for the balloon controller

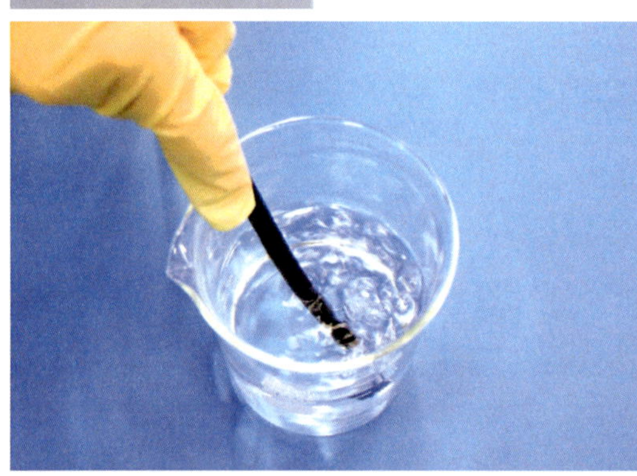

Fig. 7.4b. Check the endoscope air route for blockage

5. Press and light up the overtube selector switch (1) on the remote switch box (Fig. 7.4a) to inflate the overtube balloon. Immerse the overtube balloon in a glass of water to check it for air leaks (Fig. 7.5). After confirmation, press the overtube selector switch (1) again to turn its light off and deflate the balloon.

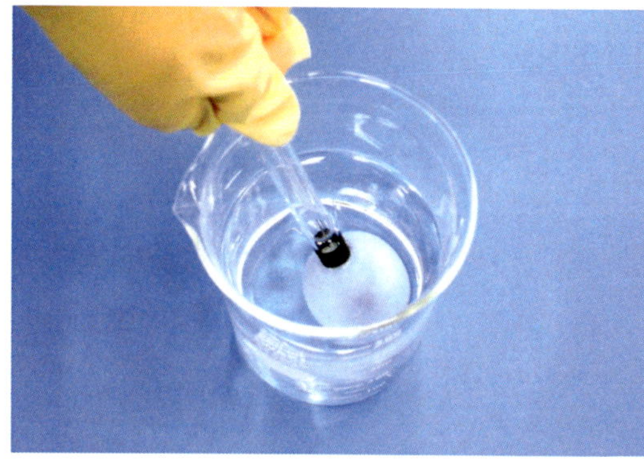

Fig. 7.5. Check the overtube balloon for air leaks

6. To lubricate the endoscope, pour 10–20 ml of water into the overtube; then hold and move the overtube to run the water through it (Fig. 7.6).

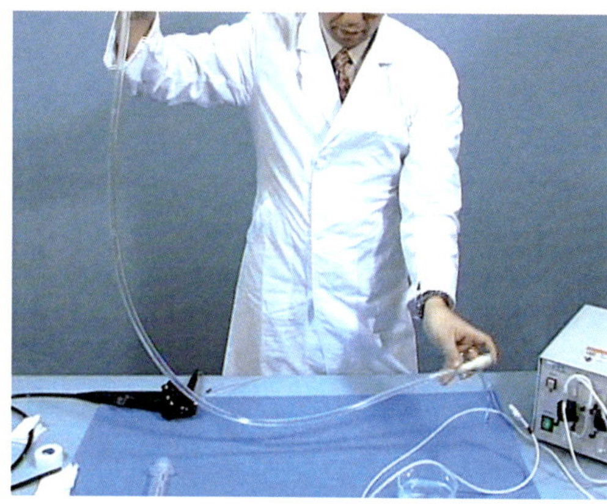

Fig. 7.6. Wet the inside of the overtube

7. Press and turn off the light of the scope pause switch (4) (Fig. 7.4a) and pass the endoscope through the overtube while air is coming out of the endoscope tip (Fig. 7.7). After the passage, slide the overtube close to the endoscope handle, wipe water off the endoscope tip, and press the scope pause switch (4).

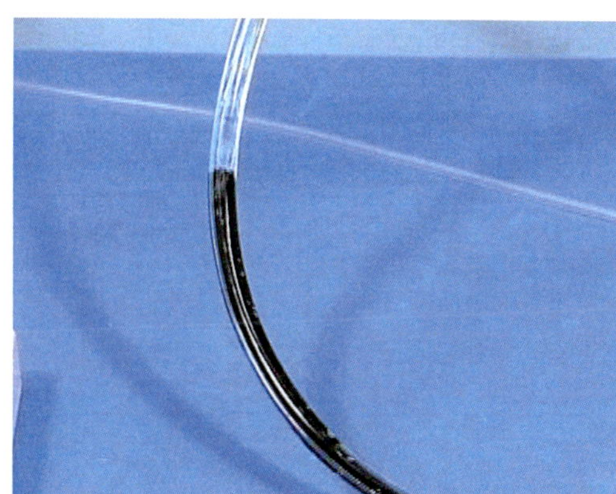

Fig. 7.7. Pass the endoscope through the overtube

8. Use an alcohol swab to wet the device used to attach a balloon to the tip (jig) and mount an endoscope balloon (Fig. 7.8).

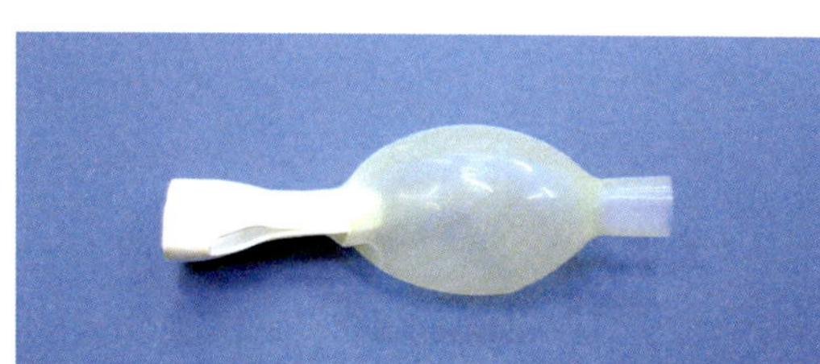

Fig. 7.8. Mount the endoscope balloon on a jig

9. Use an alcohol swab to wet the endoscope tip and attach the endoscope balloon mounted on the device (jig) onto the endoscope tip (Fig. 7.9).

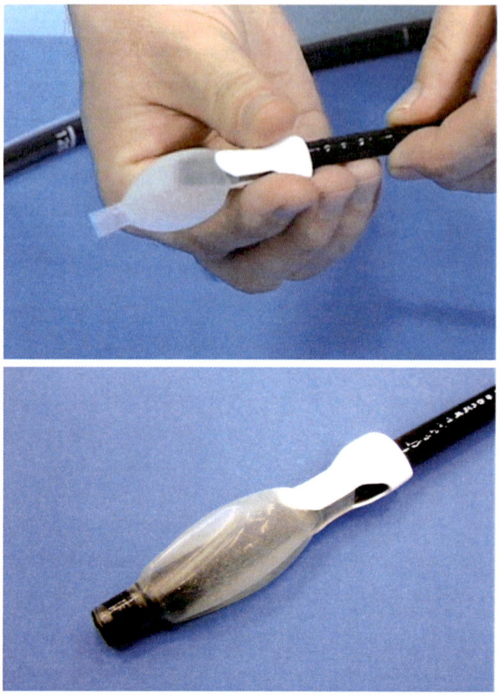

Fig. 7.9. Attach the endoscope balloon to the endoscope tip

10. Mount a fixing rubber on a mounting tool (Fig. 7.10a). Use the mounting tool to secure the endoscope balloon with the fixing rubber at a site close to the handle (Fig. 7.10b).

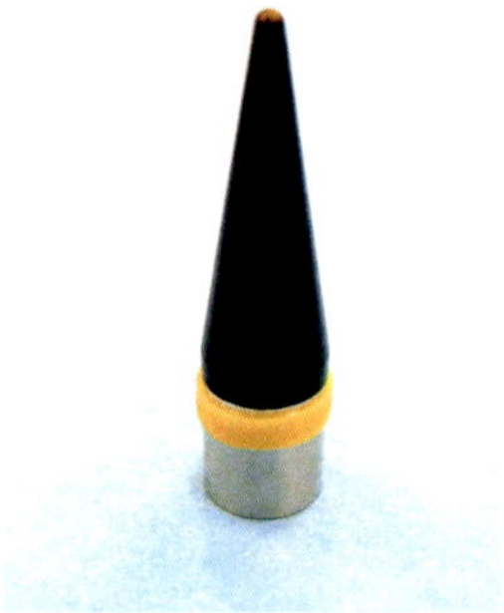

Fig. 7.10a. Mount a fixing rubber on a mounting tool

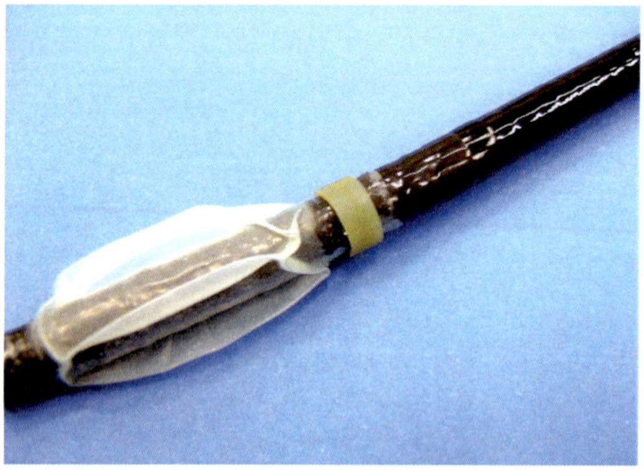

Fig. 7.10b. Secure the endoscope balloon with the fixing rubber at a site close to the handle

11. Attach a hood to the distal end of the endoscope balloon (Fig. 7.11). Watch the endoscopic monitor to ensure that the hood does not interfere with the field of view.

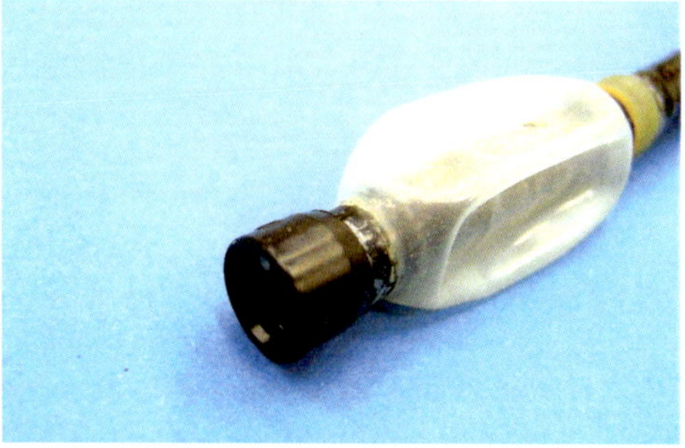

Fig. 7.11. Mount a hood

12. Cut surgical tape into a strip (width 7 mm, length 30 mm) and wind the strip around the boundary between the hood and the endoscope balloon (Fig. 7.12a). Use the mounting tool to mount the fixing rubber so the fixing rubber and the surgical tape wound on the endoscope balloon overlap (Fig. 7.12b).

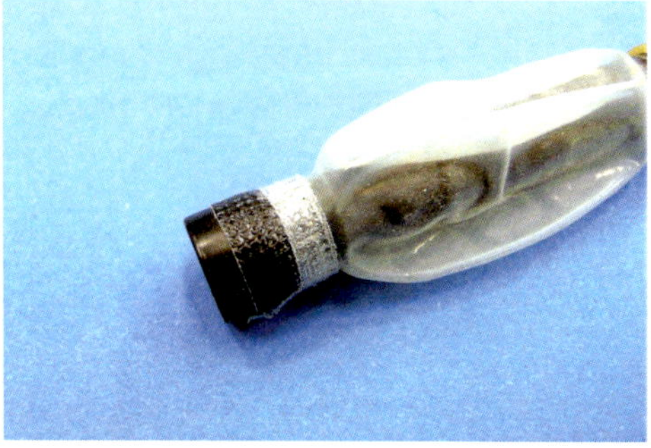

Fig. 7.12a. Wind surgical tape around the boundary between the hood and the endoscope balloon

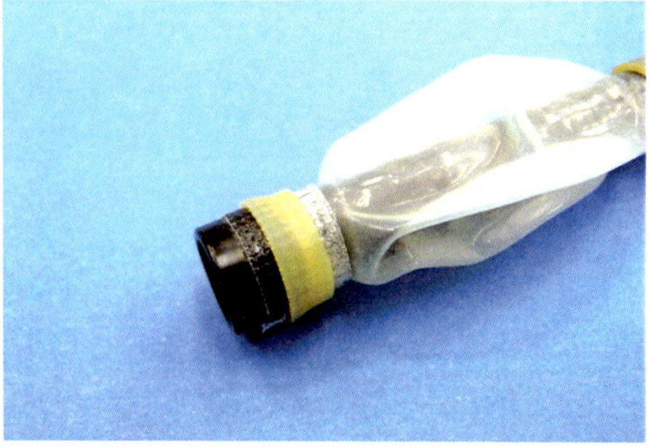

Fig. 7.12b. Use the mounting tool to mount the fixing rubber

13. Press and turn off the light of the scope pause switch (4) (Fig. 7.4a) and immerse the endoscope tip in a glass of water to examine the inflated endoscope balloon for air leaks (Fig. 7.13). Then, press and turn off the light of the scope selector switch (2) to deflate the endoscope balloon.

14. Finally, apply antifog lens cleaner to the objective lens at the endoscope tip.

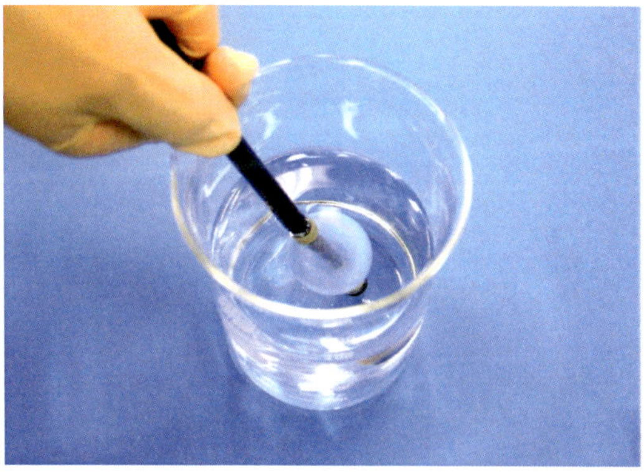

Fig. 7.13. Check the endoscope balloon for air leaks

7.2 Points to Consider About Preparation

It should be noted that two selector switches not lighting up on the controller indicate an exhaust mode (air is being withdrawn from the balloon) when the power of the balloon pump controller is turned on. In particular, if the endoscope tip is immersed in water while the scope selector switch indicates an exhaust mode, water is aspirated into the air route of the endoscope, which may block the air route. Caution should be exercised to avoid accidental water aspiration when the endoscope is withdrawn from the overtube after completing the examination. Air should be delivered whenever the endoscope tip without a balloon is immersed in water.

The balloon controller is designed to activate an alarm when abnormal balloon pressure occurs. Specifically, an alarm sounds when the air supply continues without a change in balloon pressure (if a pressure of 5.6 kPa is not achieved within 60 s of air supply or an air route pressure of 5.6 kPa is not maintained for 40 s or more during air supply) or when there is an abnormal increase in the balloon pressure (the air route pressure is 8.2 kPa or above for 5 s or more). It is desirable to press the pause switch or turn off the power of the balloon pump controller when a balloon is not firmly attached to the scope during preparation and air supply or withdrawal is not necessary. It is particularly advisable to take these precautions until you familiarize yourself with preparation procedures.

If the endoscope is removed while leaving the overtube in the intestinal tract for a certain treatment, a fixing rubber should not be used to secure the endoscope balloon (fixing rubber may stick to the overtube, which prevents removal of the endoscope). In this case, both the distal and proximal end of the endoscope balloon should be secured with nylon thread (Fig. 7.14). In principle, a hood should not be attached to the endoscope in this situation. When a hood is absolutely necessary at the time of endoscope insertion, it should be noted that the hood must be left in the intestinal tract at the time the endoscope is removed. The hood may be collected endoscopically at the end of the treatment, or it may be excreted in the feces.

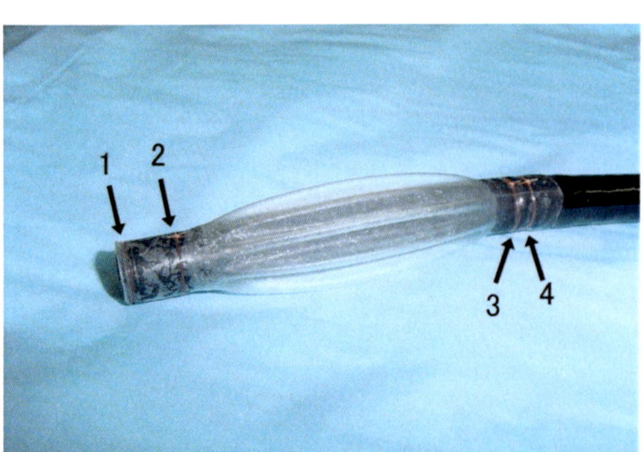

Fig. 7.14. Secure the endoscope balloon with thread. Secure the balloon at four sites. The second ligature from the tip should be placed distal to the opening of the air route. Without the second ligature, a deflated endoscope balloon may interfere with the field of view during examination

The distal end of the double-balloon endoscope has grooves where the endoscope balloon is secured with thread. Practically, two fixing rubbers are sufficient to secure the balloon, as described above; however, these grooves may be used to secure the balloon, and the following step should be taken between procedures (9) and (10).

Either nylon fishing line (approximately 0.145 mm in diameter, equivalent to no. 0.8) or nylon surgical sutures (3-0 or 4-0) are used to tie the endoscope balloon and the distal end of the endoscope together at the sites of the grooves (Figs. 7.15, 7.16).

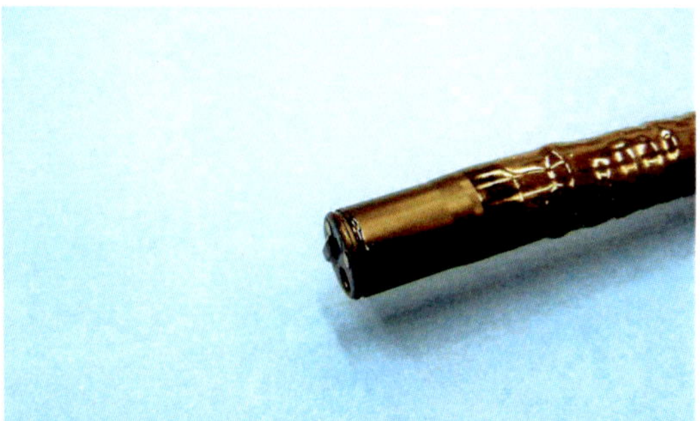

Fig. 7.15. Groove at the distal end of the endoscope

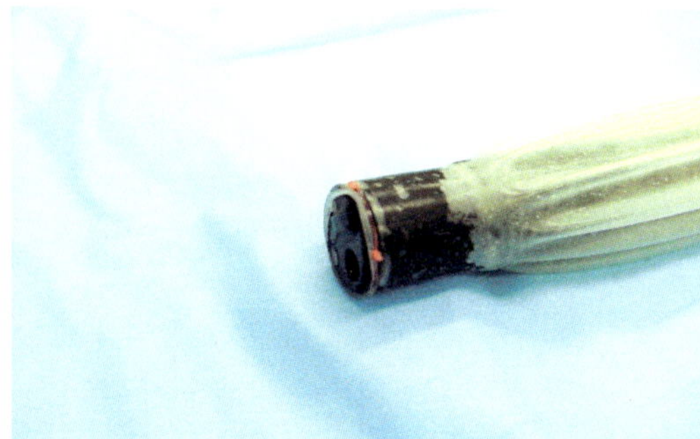

Fig. 7.16. Secure the distal end of the endoscope balloon with nylon thread

We tentatively make a knot as shown in Fig. 7.17, pass the endoscope through the knot as indicated with a star, and then tighten the knot by pulling on both ends. After making another knot, we wind the rest of the line around the endoscope and tie it again.

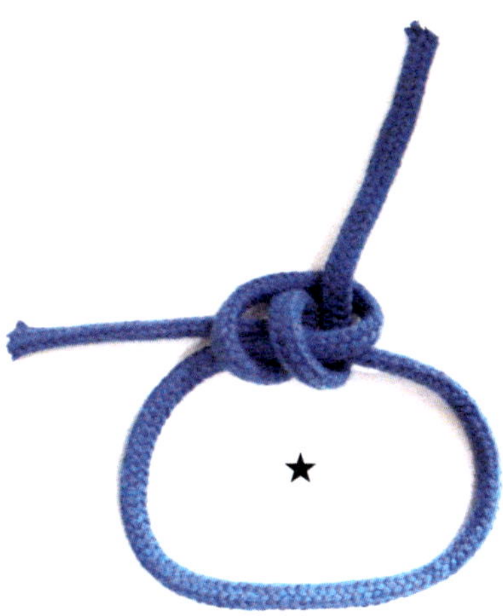

Fig. 7.17. Example of a tentative knot in nylon thread

8 Specific Procedures for Insertion

8.1 General Considerations for Endoscopy

The double-balloon endoscope can be inserted through the mouth and the anus. Before insertion procedures specific for individual approaches are detailed, considerations common to both approaches are described.

It is essential to provide the patient with adequate information on the examination and obtain informed consent before endoscopy. To relieve anxiety, the physician should inform the patient immediately before the examination that it takes more time than routine endoscopy but causes little or no pain—and that the physician is ready to treat any discomfort of which the patient complains. To monitor the patient's condition during the examination, monitors such as electrocardiography, a pulse oximeter, and an automated sphygmomanometer should be ready for use, and an intravenous line should be established to administer additional doses of sedatives.

Devices should be arranged to ensure that a fluoroscopic monitor and an endoscopic monitor can be seen simultaneously because some manipulations during the examination require simultaneous monitoring of fluoroscopic and endoscopic views. The floor preferably is covered with a water-absorbing sheet because intestinal fluids may come out of the rear end of the overtube.

A total of five buttons are used to operate the pump that controls balloons at the endoscope tip and the overtube. Air supply and withdrawal buttons, pause buttons for individual balloons and an alarm stop button are available. The pump that controls the balloons at the endoscope tip and the overtube continuously monitors the balloon pressure and automatically maintains the internal pressure of inflated balloons at a set pressure of 6 kPa (45 mm Hg). It is designed to activate an alarm when the balloon pressure exceeds the limit or fails to reach the set pressure after a certain amount of time on the air supply. Whenever an alarm sounds during the examination, its cause should be identified and the pump temporarily stopped as needed. When the balloon is inflated at a site with a large internal diameter, even a large amount of air supplied may fail to elevate the balloon pressure to a set pressure, and an alarm is activated because of an excessive amount of air supplied. Caution must be exercised because the balloon may be damaged if the problem is not addressed. Pressing the pause button is recommended to prevent balloon damage when the cause of the alarm cannot be quickly determined.

All devices should be ready for use, as described in Chapter 7. Balloons should be carefully tested to ensure that they have no air leaks and to avoid reinsertion because of balloon defects found during the examination.

Smooth insertion of the double-balloon endoscope requires techniques for advancing the endoscope tip with a minimum of force. That is because endoscope insertion is based on a point supported by the overtube balloon, and the support by the balloon is kept to a minimum to ensure safety. Forcible insertion does not advance the endoscope tip but only withdraws the overtube. This is required to ensure safety, and only the allowable range of insertion force should be applied to advance the endoscope tip smoothly.

Specifically, forcible insertion of a sharply angled endoscope should be avoided. The operator should insert the endoscope while reducing the angle as much as possible and swinging the tip so the endoscope forms a large arc.

Air insufflation during insertion should be kept to a minimum. This is important for keeping the patient's discomfort to a minimum and for pleating the intestine over the overtube. To keep air insufflation to a minimum and negotiate bends using a slalom technique during insertion, we usually insert the endoscope with a hood attached to its tip. This hood prevents "red-out" and facilitates insertion by the slalom technique with a minimum of air insufflation.

Because insertion of the double-balloon endoscope is based on the grip of the intestine by the balloon, the operator advances the endoscope or the overtube only after confirming that the balloon is adequately inflated or deflated. A balloon is considered to be inflated enough to have a good grip when the pressure gauge of the pump indicates a stable level of 6 kPa. A balloon is considered to be adequately deflated when the pump stops making an air-withdrawal sound.

In principle, the double-balloon endoscope is inserted with concomitant monitoring of the shape of the endoscope and the condition of the balloon with a fluoroscope as needed; however, experienced physicians do not need frequent use of a fluoroscope. The duration of fluoroscopy should be minimized to keep the extent of exposure to a minimum.

Both balloons (at the endoscope tip and the overtube) are initially deflated; and the overtube is placed at the rear end of the endoscope so the portion of the endoscope beyond the tip of the overtube is as long as possible. The operator should hold the endoscope tip for insertion without the aid of an assistant. When the overtube is inserted, the assistant stands between the operator and the patient to hold the overtube straight and insert it along the endoscope. The inner and outer surface of the overtube is coated with hydrophilic material, and lubricity between the overtube and the endoscope is improved by injecting water into the overtube. Thus, the assistant injects water as needed.

A 155-cm marking on the endoscope can be used as a guide, and the overtube is inserted until its rear end reaches the marking. When the rear end reaches that position, the tip of the overtube reaches the proximity of the balloon attached to the endoscope tip. During the examination, bear in mind that further insertion may cause interference of the tip of the overtube with the balloon at the endoscope tip, dislocation of the balloon, or damage to the balloon. Although the clearance between the tip of the overtube and the endoscope is kept to a minimum, the intestinal wall could become entangled in the clearance when the intestine is sharply angled. When abnormal resistance occurs during insertion of the overtube, the cause should be determined fluoroscopically instead of by forcible insertion. Any sharp bend should be reduced by withdrawing the endoscope and reinserting the overtube. Because the overtube is inserted without fluoroscopic guidance, it is important to insert the overtube gently to prevent it from catching the intestinal mucosa. When insertion of the overtube is difficult, a jiggling technique may facilitate insertion.

After inserting the overtube, the assistant holds the overtube on the portion outside of the body with both hands: The overtube close to the insertion site of the patient (mouth or anus) is held with the left hand, and the rear end of the overtube is held with the right hand, with the result that the overtube is held in a straightened position between the two hands. The operator manipulates the endoscope as he or she inserts it into the rear end of the overtube, so the assistant should hold the rear end of the overtube securely (Fig. 8.1). For double-balloon endoscopy, not only the operator but also the assistant should be familiar with the principle of insertion and notable complications.

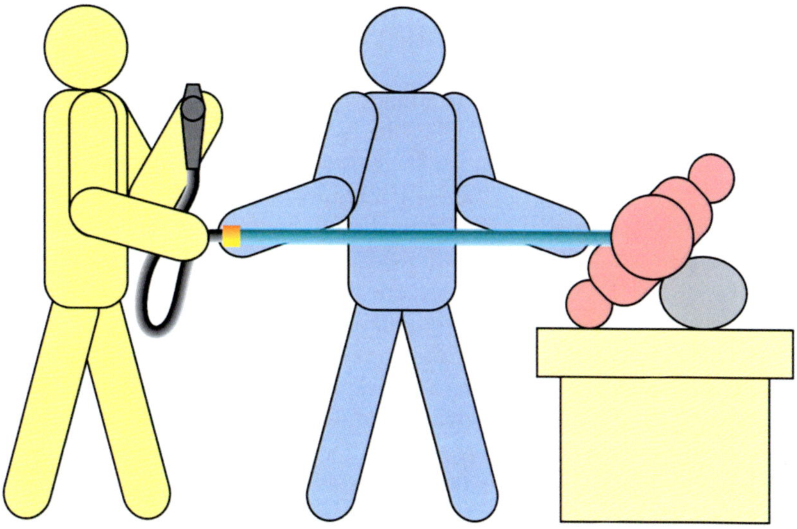

Fig. 8.1. Operator, assistant, and patient

8.2 Insertion Through the Mouth (Anterograde Approach)

Before starting the oral insertion, a lubricant (such as Xylocaine jelly) is applied to the distal end of the endoscope (including the balloon). As in the case of upper gastrointestinal endoscopy, a mouthpiece is used. The endoscope is advanced into the stomach without the aid of an assistant, as in the case of conventional upper gastrointestinal endoscopy. Unlike the conventional upper gastrointestinal endoscope, the thin, flexible endoscope tends to bend in the mouth, and it is rather difficult to transmit the force to the endoscope tip. Another difference is that the endoscope between the two hands tends to trail down because of its long total length. These two issues can be addressed by inserting the overtube along the endoscope with the assistant holding the overtube; therefore, attention is given to these issues only during the initial phase of insertion.

When the endoscope tip is advanced into the stomach, gastric contents are suctioned well to prevent aspiration during the examination and unnecessary looping in the stomach. Air insufflation should be kept to a minimum, and the endoscope tip is advanced to the gastric antrum.

At this stage, the assistant stands between the operator and the patient to insert the overtube along the endoscope while straightening the overtube. The overtube is inserted with the balloon at the endoscope tip deflated because inflation of the balloon in the stomach may damage the balloon. Because insertion through the mouth causes the greatest discomfort to the patient when the endoscope and the overtube advance beyond the larynx, application of adequate lubricant jelly is necessary at the time of the initial insertion of the endoscope as well as insertion of the overtube. Manipulation of the endoscope without movement of the overtube causes no irritation in the larynx, but manipulation of the overtube may irritate the larynx and cause discomfort to the patient. Thus, the overtube should be gently manipulated with particular attention paid to this point.

After the rear end of the overtube reaches the 155-cm marking on the endoscope, the endoscope tip is advanced into the descending or horizontal part of the duodenum with the overtube balloon deflated, after which the balloon at the endoscope tip is inflated. The overtube is inserted along the endoscope until the rear end of the overtube reaches the 155-cm marking on the endoscope; then the overtube balloon is inflated to secure the tip of the overtube in the duodenum. When it is difficult to insert the overtube, pulling back and straightening the endoscope may facilitate insertion, as in the case of conventional upper gastrointestinal endoscopy.

The tip of the overtube may not be secured in the duodenum and may slip back into the stomach. One can estimate whether it is successfully secured on the basis of the condition of the air supply from the pump. A small volume of air allows the internal pressure of the balloon in the duodenum to reach the set pressure, and the pump automatically stops supplying air. When the balloon is in the stomach, however, even a large volume of air may fail to elevate the balloon pressure, and an alarm is activated. In such cases, the pump should be stopped temporarily because continued air supply from the pump may damage the balloon. In this case, there should be no further attempts to secure the tip of the overtube in the duodenum at this stage. Instead, the balloon at the endoscope tip is deflated, and the endoscope is pushed into the deeper portion of the duodenum. Then the balloon at the endoscope tip is inflated, the overtube is advanced again, and the tip of the overtube is secured in the duodenum.

After the endoscope and the overtube are withdrawn with both balloons inflated to reduce looping in the stomach, the balloon at the endoscope tip is deflated, and the endoscope is advanced beyond the ligament of Treitz. During the process, the tip of the overtube is secured in the duodenum, which allows deep insertion of the endoscope without loops in the stomach.

The endoscope is advanced as far as possible, and the balloon at the endoscope tip is inflated and secured in the intestine. Then the overtube balloon is deflated, and the overtube is inserted along the endoscope. After the overtube balloon is inflated again and secured in the intestine, both the endoscope and the overtube are pulled back slowly with both balloons inflated to eliminate redundant loops, followed by deflation of the balloon at the endoscope tip and insertion of the endoscope. These procedures are repeated to advance the endoscope while the fixed support established by the overtube balloon is moved more deeply (Fig. 8.2).

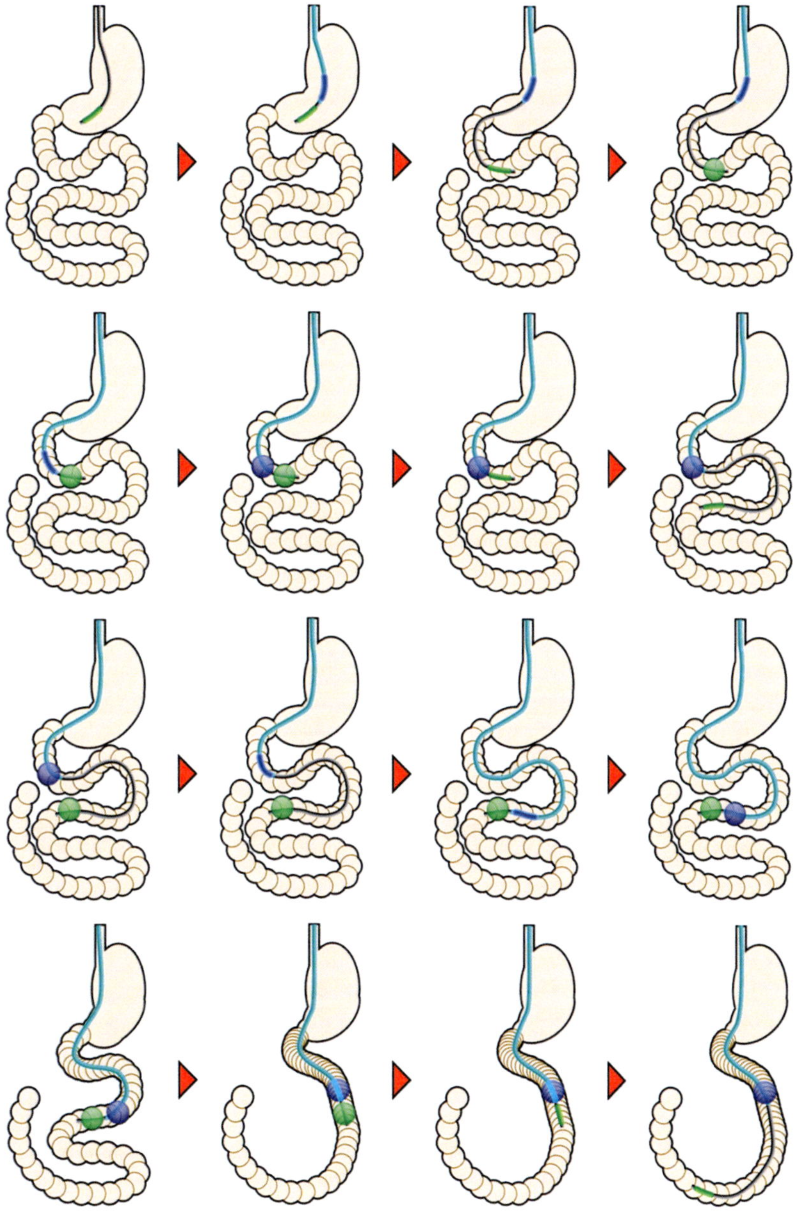

Fig. 8.2. Insertion through the mouth

8.3 Insertion Through the Anus (Retrograde Approach)

Initially with anal insertion, the operator holds the endoscope tip with the right hand and starts inserting it without the aid of an assistant, similar to conventional colonoscopy. Unlike conventional colonoscopy, it is not necessary to try to insert the endoscope straight from the rectum to the sigmoid colon. After the endoscope is inserted about 50 cm and the tip of the overtube is positioned close to the anus, the balloon at the endoscope tip is inflated, and the overtube is inserted along the endoscope. The overtube is inserted until its rear end reaches the 155-cm marking on the endoscope, and then the overtube balloon is inflated so both balloons grip the intestine. Slow withdrawal of the endoscope and the overtube with both balloons inflated allows easy reduction of loops because the distal ends are secured by the balloons. If it is difficult to straighten the sigmoid colon because of adhesions or other reasons, proceed to the next step without making further efforts to straighten the colon.

After overtube insertion, the assistant holds the portion of the overtube that is outside the body in a straightened position. The operator manipulates the endoscope as he or she inserts it to the rear end of the overtube. After the balloon at the endoscope tip is deflated, the endoscope is advanced as far as possible, and the balloon at the endoscope tip is then inflated to secure the endoscope in the intestine. Thereafter, the overtube balloon is deflated, and the overtube is advanced along the endoscope until it reaches the balloon at the endoscope tip. These procedures are repeated, thereby advancing the endoscope while the fixed support established by the overtube balloon is moved from the sigmoid–descending colon junction to the splenic flexure or the hepatic flexure (Fig. 8.3). In cases where insertion is easy, direct insertion into the splenic flexure and positioning the balloon in the splenic flexure may allow further insertion into the cecum. In most cases, the passage through the large intestine requires one to three sessions of balloon manipulation.

During the procedures, attention should be given to the following points: Because the large intestine has a greater internal diameter than the small intestine, an alarm may be activated during balloon inflation if the balloon pressure fails to reach the set pressure and the pump continues to supply air beyond the allowed inflation time. The pump should be stopped temporarily because continued air supply may damage the balloon. In this case, although the balloon pressure is below the set pressure, the balloon is inflated enough to grip the intestine. The operator may therefore proceed to the next step while the pump is stopped temporarily.

When it is difficult to advance the endoscope tip beyond the ileocecal valve, the overtube should be slightly pulled back, with the balloon inflated in the ascending colon. This manipulation allows the ileocecal region to form an obtuse angle (Fig. 8.4) and facilitates insertion into the ileum. After the endoscope is advanced as far as possible beyond the ileocecal valve, the balloon at the endoscope tip is inflated, the overtube balloon is deflated, and the overtube is then inserted along the endoscope. The tip of the overtube is presumably advanced beyond the ileocecal valve when the pump stops automatically within a short period of time because the ileum is much narrower than the large intestine, requiring only a small volume of air to inflate the balloon. In the next step, if the pump resumes applying air during further insertion of the endoscope into the ileum with its balloon deflated, the overtube balloon placed in the ileum is likely to have slipped from the ileum to the large intestine. If excess air supply makes the pump activate an alarm, the pump should be paused temporarily and endoscope insertion continued. In principle, the endoscope should be inserted into the distal small intestine after the overtube is pulled back enough to pleat the intestine over the overtube, as described later. When the overtube is barely advanced into the ileum, however, the overtube balloon tends to slip to the cecum. Thus, the endoscope should be inserted without excess pullback of the overtube. It is important to avoid excess twisting of the endoscope tip in the ileum and to advance the endoscope so it naturally forms concentric circles. It should be noted that insertion of a twisted endoscope downward results in sigmoidal insertion in the direction of the pelvis, which makes further insertion difficult.

It should be noted also that, unlike insertion through the mouth, insertion through the anus is opposite in direction to intestinal peristalsis. Care should therefore be taken to suppress intestinal peristalsis because the peristalsis pushes the balloon backward.

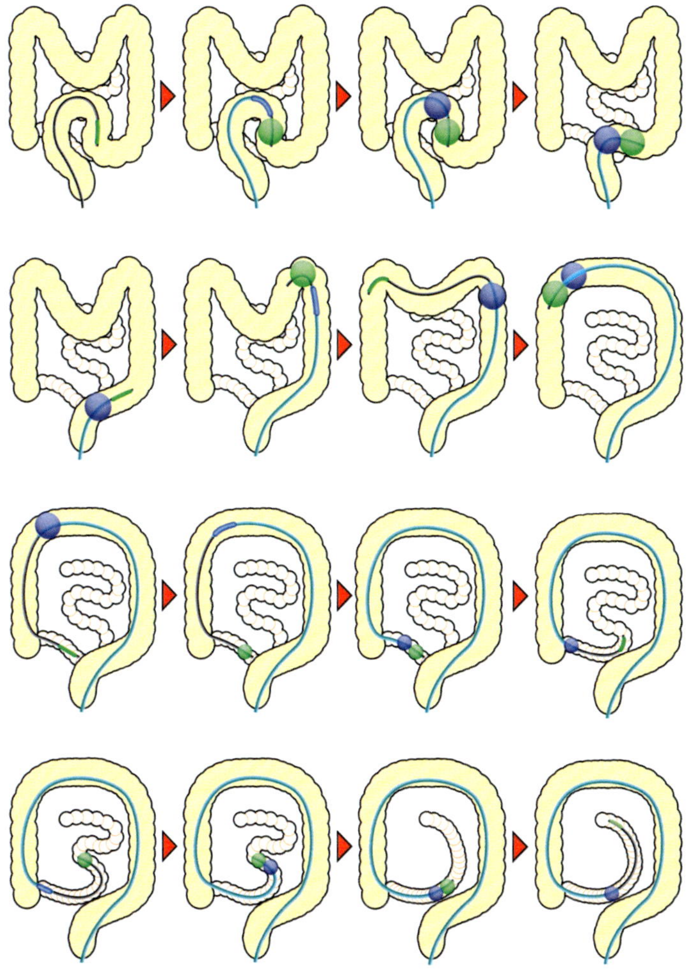

Fig. 8.3. Insertion through the anus

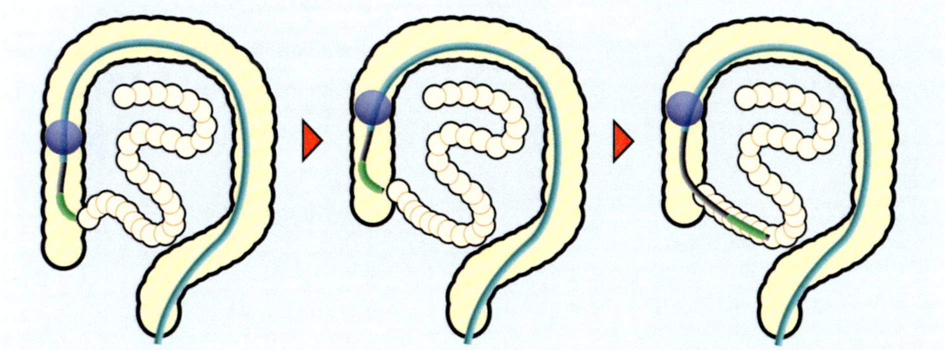

Fig. 8.4. Widening of the angulated ileocecal region

8.4 Manipulation in the Distal Small Intestine

The basic insertion technique for the distal small intestine is to advance the endoscope tip with minimum insertion force so the endoscope forms large concentric circles (which are formed by stretching the mesentery in a fan shape around the fixed part of the mesentery on the retroperitoneum) (Figs. 8.5, 8.6). As described above, the operator should avoid forcible insertion of a sharply angled endoscope. Reducing the angle as much as possible and swinging the tip allows effective insertion. The small intestine is freely mobile, and its bends are not fixed unless there are adhesions. It is therefore unnecessary to intricately bend the endoscope to follow the bends ahead. Small turns are negotiable by changing the direction of the endoscope tip and using the slalom technique. After the endoscope is inserted until its proximal end reaches the rear end of the overtube, the balloon at the endoscope tip is inflated to secure the endoscope tip at this position, the overtube balloon is deflated, and the overtube is inserted along the endoscope. After the rear end of the overtube reaches the 155-cm marking on the endoscope, the overtube balloon is inflated so both balloons can grip the intestine. With both balloons inflated, the endoscope is withdrawn together with the overtube to pleat the intestine over the overtube and to shorten it.

During the procedures the operator may use fluoroscopic images to ensure that the entire endoscope forms concentric circles (continuous fluoroscopic monitoring is not necessary for experienced operators) and endoscopic views to ensure that the balloons are in position. The small intestine is freely mobile in the abdominal cavity. When the endoscope seemingly slips on a fluoroscopic image but not on an endoscopic view, the endoscope is actually in position, and the small intestine is changing position instead. This manipulation reduces looping without the endoscope tip slipping, and it gathers and shortens the inserted intestine on the overtube. The manipulation not only shortens the intestine to make the best use of the working length of the endoscope, it also straightens the intestine ahead and reduces

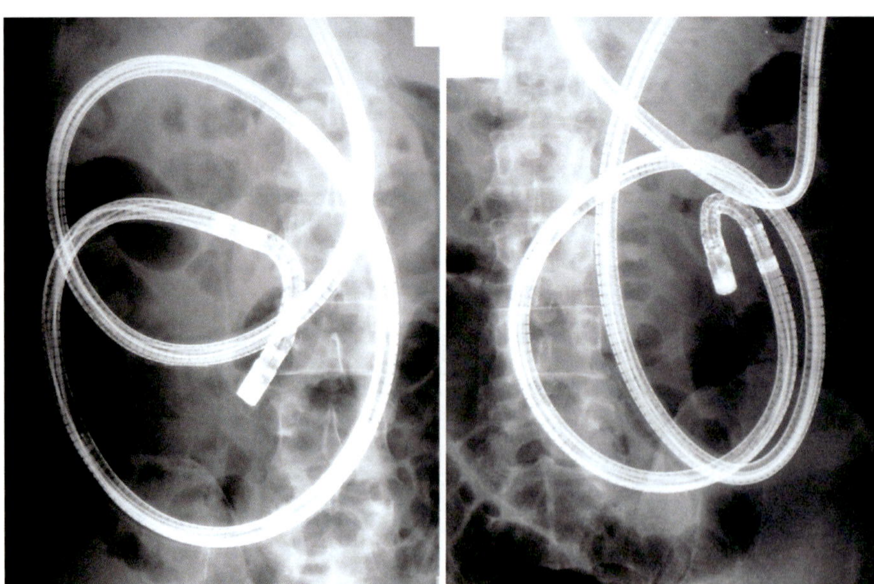

Fig. 8.5. Concentric insertion (through the mouth)

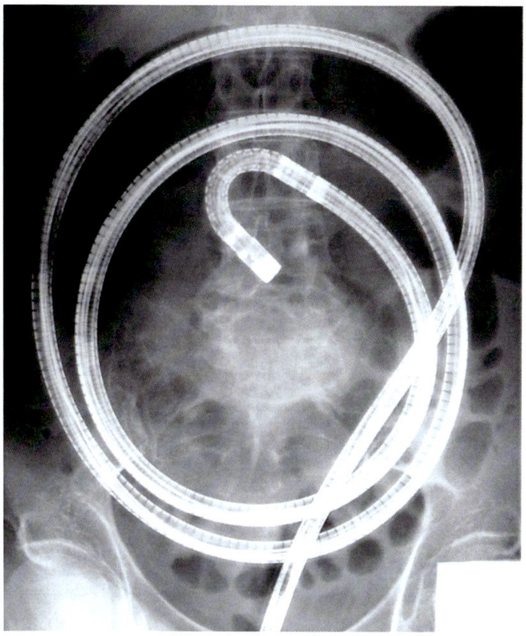

Fig. 8.6. Concentric insertion (through the anus)

bends, thereby facilitating insertion. Once the intestine adopts a shape that facilitates effective insertion, the endoscope tip can be advanced by repeating the endoscope insertion and shortening of the small intestine, with the shape maintained. The endoscope tip is actually advancing even when it seemingly moves back and forth on a fluoroscopic monitor.

When a sharp bend makes insertion difficult, the overtube is advanced to the bend instead of trying forcible insertion. Both balloons are then inflated to grip the intestine, and the endoscope is withdrawn together with the overtube to reduce the bend, which facilitates insertion. In short, double-balloon endoscopy makes use of the mobility of the small intestine and allows insertion while modifying the shape of the intestine for easy insertion. This should be kept in mind to achieve efficient insertion.

When inserted through the mouth, the endoscope may be advanced clockwise or counterclockwise to the patient so long as it allows smooth insertion (Fig. 8.5). When inserted through the anus, the endoscope should be inserted to ensure that it forms concentric circles counterclockwise (Fig. 8.6). Concentric insertion facilitates shortening of the small intestine and allows good maneuverability of the endoscope tip.

Nonconcentric insertion may be addressed by withdrawing the endoscope and overtube with the balloons inflated as much as possible before slipping or adjusting the direction of the endoscope tip under fluoroscopic guidance. For insertion through the anus, the ileum adjacent to the ileocecal region may be positioned deep in the pelvic cavity, precluding concentric insertion. In this case, fluoroscopy is used to drag out the ileum lying deep down to ensure concentric insertion. The small intestine is freely mobile unless there is an adhesion in the abdominal cavity, and it is therefore possible to adjust the shape and position of the small intestine to facilitate endoscope insertion. The concentric shape is favorable for physiological movement of intestinal contents, and repositioning the small intestine has caused no problem in patients.

After deep insertion into the small intestine and inflation of the balloon at the endoscope tip, further insertion of the overtube may be impossible because most of the overtube is inserted in the body with a minimal part on the outside (Fig. 8.7). At this stage, the balloon at the endoscope tip is inflated, and the overtube is withdrawn together with the endoscope before the overtube balloon is deflated. After the endoscope is withdrawn until the 155-cm marking comes out of the body, the overtube balloon is deflated, and the overtube is inserted along the endoscope (Fig. 8.8A). If only the endoscope is withdrawn and the overtube is not pulled back, subsequent insertion will be less effective. Withdrawal of the endoscope alone shortens the intestine between the two balloons on the endoscope. The shortened intestine remains between the two balloons after the overtube is advanced and its balloon is inflated. When the balloon at the endoscope tip is deflated, the shortened intestine instantly stretches beyond the endoscope tip, precluding effective insertion (Fig. 8.8B).

The endoscope tip in the distal small intestine is most likely to slip when the small intestine is shortened with both balloons inflated and the balloon at the endoscope tip is deflated. The operator should be alert and ready to advance the endoscope when deflating the balloon at the endoscope tip in the distal small intestine.

When endoscope insertion is difficult and reaches a deadlock, the posture of the patient can be changed. This may break the deadlock because a change in the influence of gravity may alter the positional relation between the intestine and the endoscope in the abdominal cavity and the distribution of intestinal contents.

Although the double-balloon method allows total enteroscopy, insertion efficiency decreases in the distal small intestine because the length of advancement for each balloon manipulation is shorter as the endoscope is advanced more deeply. Insertion via the mouth into the ileocecal region is possible under favorable conditions. However, it is more efficient to perform two examinations: one through the mouth and the other through the anus. When two examinations are performed, a tattoo is placed at the deepest reachable point, which is used as a mark during the subsequent examination from the opposite direction. Whether the endoscope is to be inserted through the mouth or the anus during the initial examination is carefully determined on the basis of the patient's medical history and the

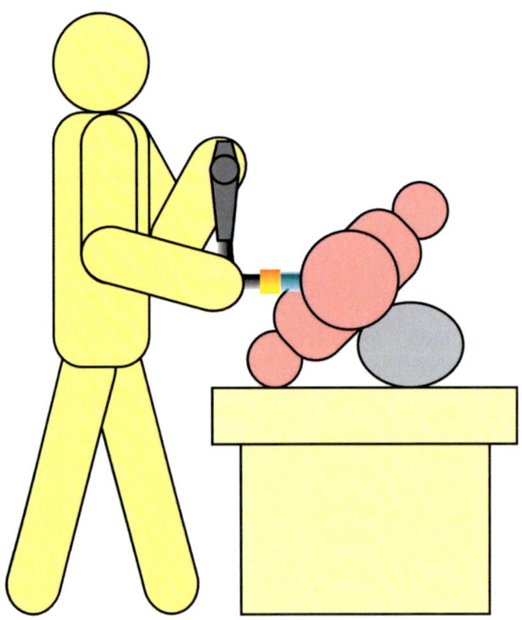

Fig. 8.7. Condition that precludes overtube insertion

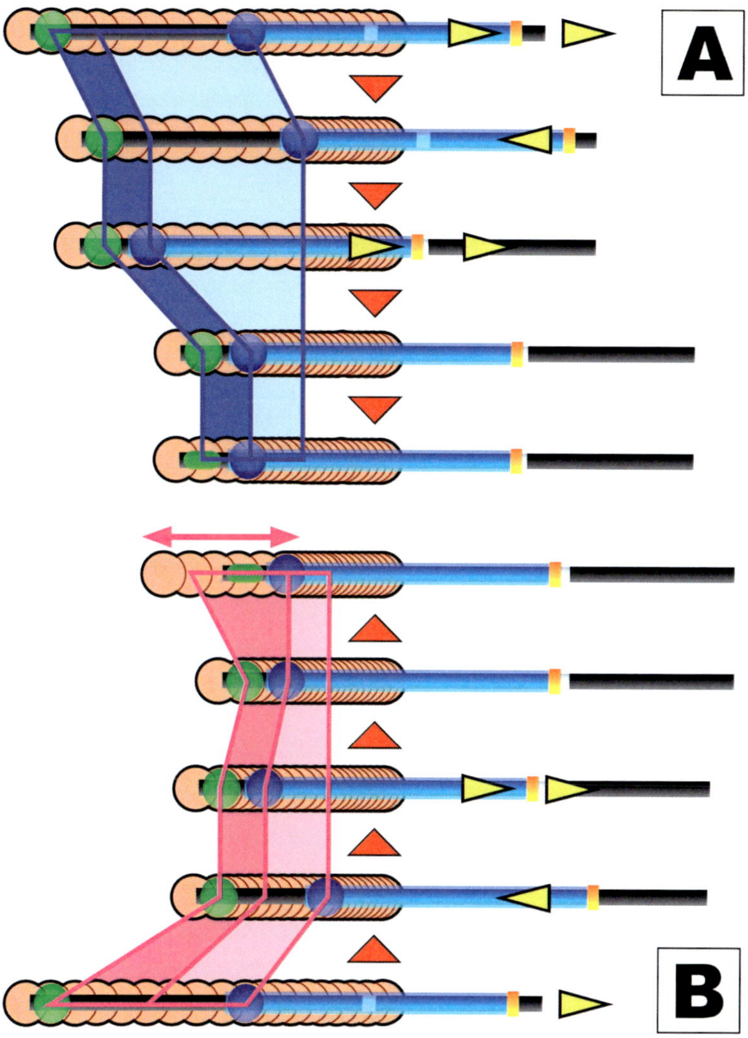

Fig. 8.8.A,B. It is more effective when the overtube is withdrawn together with the endoscope. **A** Effective shortening is achieved by withdrawing both the overtube and the endoscope. **B** Shortening by withdrawing the endoscope alone results in less effective insertion

results of the preoperative examination; however, a lack of information for decision making is not uncommon. When total enteroscopy is indicated, we preferentially insert the endoscope through the anus because this method causes less discomfort to the patient. We observe the widest possible area by anal insertion, thereby reducing the time of observation required with the oral insertion. Unless an emergency dictates otherwise, examination from the opposite direction is preferably performed on some other day because of concerns about residual air entering the intestinal tract during endoscopic observation.

9 Expected Complications and Procedures to Address the Complications

The double-balloon endoscope can be inserted through the mouth or the anus, and due caution should be exercised because these approaches may cause complications similar to those associated with conventional upper and lower gastrointestinal endoscopy. Double-balloon endoscopy allows observation of the distal small intestine not accessible by conventional endoscopy; however, it inevitably prolongs the examination time, and thus it is desirable to monitor blood pressure, oxygen saturation, and the electrocardiogram during examination. Because double-balloon endoscopy differs from conventional endoscopy regarding its indications, observation range, and the use of an overtube and balloons, the potential risk of additional complications should be taken into consideration. This chapter describes complications specific to double-balloon endoscopy and the procedures that can be used to address those complications.

9.1 Complications Related to Specific Indications

Double-balloon endoscopy permits insertion of the endoscope into regions not accessible to the conventional endoscope and allows endoscopic diagnosis of lesions in the distal small intestine that was previously impossible. Because of the dramatic increase in the observable area, endoscopy is considered for disorders in which conventional endoscopy is not indicated. However, criteria for performing conventional endoscopy may not be relevant to double-balloon endoscopy, which requires careful consideration.

We experienced a patient with a malignant lymphoma of the small intestine diagnosed by double-balloon endoscopy, who required emergency surgery after follow-up double-balloon endoscopy, which revealed covered perforations in the involved region caused by the chemotherapy. Before examination, indication of the examination should be carefully evaluated considering the various risks.

9.2 Complications Related to the Overtube

There is a slight clearance between the tip of the overtube and the endoscope. Although clearance is diminished by the tapered tip of the overtube, it is increased on the outside of the sharp bend, and entanglement of the intestine and mucosal damage could occur when a sharply angled overtube is advanced. To minimize the risk, the overtube should be advanced after a sharply angled endoscope is corrected (when possible). When abnormal resistance occurs during advancement of the overtube, the condition should be monitored fluoroscopically instead of attempting forcible insertion. Any sharp bend should be reduced, after which the overtube can be further advanced.

9.3 Complications Related to Balloons

For double-balloon endoscopy, balloons used to grip the intestine are made of latex, and its inflation and deflation are controlled by an electric pump. The pump is set to maintain the internal pressure of the inflated balloon at 6.0 kPa (approximately 45 mm Hg). At that pressure, no perforation occurs in normal intestines, and the patient does not sense the presence of the balloon. However, it might cause a perforation in an intestine with deep ulcers.

It is particularly risky to insert the endoscope beyond lesions with new, deep ulcers because the balloon is inflated outside the endoscopic view. The operator should fully understand the potential risk of perforation when inserting the endoscope beyond those lesions. Inserting the overtube together with the endoscope beyond lesions is associated with an increased risk of damage to the lesions as well as perforation, requiring judgment about the need for such insertion only after carefully considering the risks.

9.4 Complications Related to Intraperitoneal Adhesions

Making use of the free mobility of the small intestine in the abdominal cavity, double-balloon endoscopy reduces bends and shortens the small intestine for insertion; however, intraperitoneal adhesions may restrict the mobility of the small intestine and make insertion difficult. In such cases, forcible manipulation of the endoscope without consideration of adhesions incurs the risk of perforation. Postural change, manual pressure, or repositioning the fixed support established by the balloon at the tip of the overtube should be considered for insertion without forcible manipulation or pushing.

9.5 Complications Associated with Selective Contrast-Enhanced Radiography

Selected contrast-enhanced studies are performed by injecting a contrast agent through the forceps channel of the double-balloon endoscope, with the balloon at the endoscope tip inflated. This allows contrast-enhanced studies in the small intestine, as well as cholangiography or pancreatography in the presence of cholangiojejunal or pancreatojejunal anastomosis. Patients undergoing pancreatography should be closely followed up because pancreatitis may occur after a routine examination. When a contrast-enhanced study is performed with the endoscope inserted through the anus into the upper jejunum, a contrast agent may regurgitate beyond the ligament of Treitz, and the stimulus may make the patient vomit. Because examining a patient in a supine position risks aspiration, a contrast-enhanced study should be performed only after preparations have been made to institute prompt measures for treating such an eventuality, including the availability of an oral suction device and postural change to a lateral position.

9.6 Complications Associated with Endoscopic Treatment

Double-balloon endoscopy enables reliable manipulation of the endoscope even in the distal small intestine, and it allows endoscopic treatments such as endoscopic hemostasis and dilatation of a stenosis. It is, however, important to understand the thinness and fragility of the intestinal wall, and perforation and other complications due to forcible manipulation should be avoided.

When coagulation procedures are performed with high-frequency current, thick tissues such as tumors may coagulate without injection. In general, however, it is safe to coagulate tissues in combination with submucosal injection.

Dilatation should be avoided for stenosis if there is an acute inflammation or ulcers, and the expansion diameter should be kept to a minimum. It is not necessary to dilate the stenosis all at once: Endoscopic dilatation can be repeated as needed.

10 Endoscopic Diagnosis

10.1 Diagnosis

10.1.1 Endoscopic Observation

Points to consider for observation with the double-balloon endoscope are described in this chapter. There is no significant difference between an observation with the double-balloon endoscope and a conventional endoscopic observation; however, air insufflation must be kept to a minimum because the double-balloon endoscope is inserted while the intestine is shortened. Thus, observation is inevitably limited during insertion, with a detailed examination being performed during removal. The examination during removal takes place while the shortened intestine is being returned to its original condition. Balloons are used to anchor the intestine during observation to prevent instant stretching of the shortened intestine and to allow observation with minimal blind spots.

More specifically, observation is started from the deepest reachable point with the overtube balloon inflated and the endoscope balloon deflated. The observation is performed while a modest amount of air is insufflated. The observation is made while the endoscope is being withdrawn up to the point at which the 155-cm marking on the endoscope reaches the rear end of the overtube (where the endoscope balloon reaches the tip of the overtube). The endoscope cannot be withdrawn further, and the endoscope balloon is then inflated to secure the endoscope temporarily at that location. Under these conditions, the overtube balloon is deflated, and the overtube alone is withdrawn approximately 10 cm (up to the 165-cm marking on the endoscope). During this manipulation, it is important not to withdraw the overtube to the proximal end of the endoscope at once. That is because the intestine is substantially shortened over the overtube during observation and because a 10-cm length of shortened intestine during withdrawal may be equivalent to a 30- to 40-cm portion of the small intestine at the time of insertion. After the overtube is withdrawn approximately 10 cm, the overtube balloon is inflated again to secure the overtube in the intestine. The endoscope balloon is deflated, and observation is made again until the 155-cm marking on the endoscope reaches the rear end of the overtube. Similar observations are repeated whenever the overtube is withdrawn approximately 10 cm. Thus, holding the intestine with the overtube balloon during withdrawal allows back-and-forth observation at any point in the distal small intestine and detailed endoscopic observation.

During this examination of the small intestine, attention should be given to villous changes. Inflammation-related erythematous or edematous villi are often found around ulcers and erosions, and the presence or absence of these findings is useful for differentiation from mucosal damage due to insertion of the endoscope (Fig. 10.1.1). Villous atrophy is often found in the mucosa of a submucosal tumor, and localized villous atrophy may be an indication of a submucosal tumor (Fig. 10.1.2). Although rare in Japan, extensive villous atrophy is observed in patients with celiac disease and other malabsorption syndromes. Because of the presence of villi in the small intestine, it is often difficult to clearly identify small areas of angiodysplasia compared with that in the large intestine, and careful observation is needed not to overlook the lesion.

Also in the small intestine, dye spraying is useful for detailed observation of lesions such as ulcers and tumors (Figs. 10.1.1, 10.1.3). Underwater observations and magnified observations are useful for detailed examination of villi (Figs. 10.1.1, 10.1.2, 10.1.4).

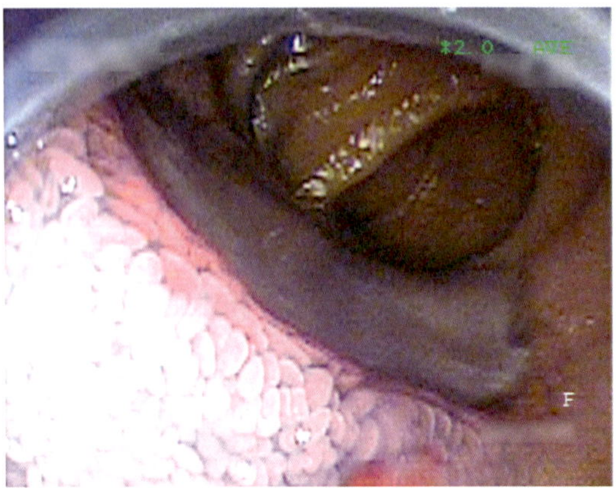

Fig. 10.1.1. Erythematous and edematous villi around the ulcer

Electronic magnified image after indigo carmine spraying

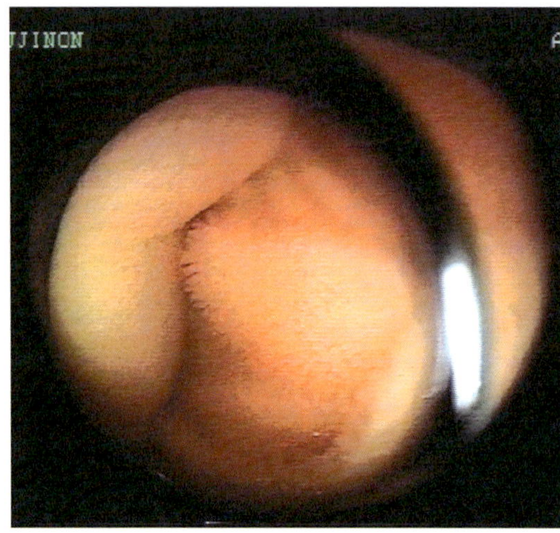

Fig. 10.1.2. Villous atrophy on a submucosal tumor (underwater examination)

Normal villi are seen in the center of the screen, and villous atrophy on the submucosal tumor is noted on the left of the screen

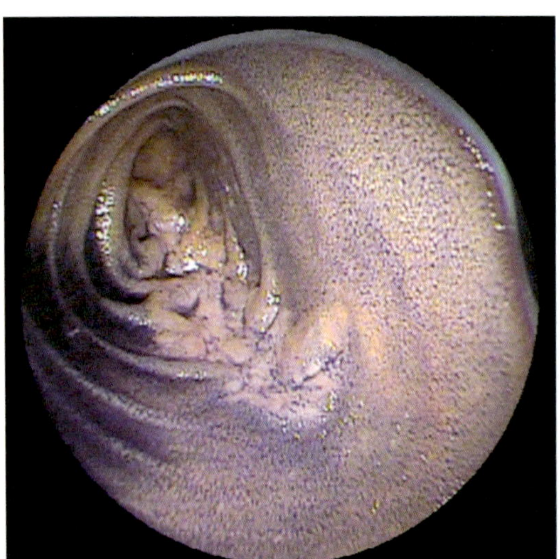

Fig. 10.1.3. Endoscopic view of mucosa-associated lymphoid tissue (MALT) lymphoma of the ileum

Indigo carmine spraying allows detailed observation of the surface

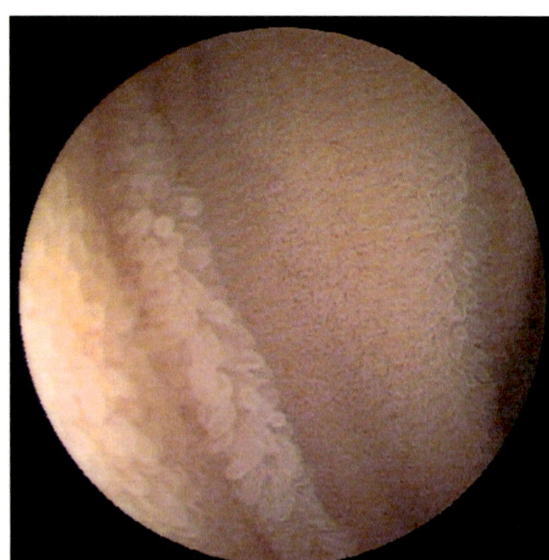

Fig. 10.1.4. Normal villi of the ileum (underwater examination)

10.1.2 Biopsy

Providing excellent maneuverability even in the distal small intestine, double-balloon endoscopy allows easily directed biopsy of localized lesions and a definitive diagnosis by pathology examination. Pathology examination of biopsy specimens of the small-intestinal mucosa should be considered also in patients with malabsorption and protein loss.

10.1.3 Topographic Diagnosis

Whether a lesion is located on the mesenteric side or the opposite side is an important clue in the differential diagnosis of intestinal diseases; previously it could be determined only after surgical findings were available and surgical specimens obtained. Using double-balloon endoscopy, it is now possible without having to resort to surgery. When the double-balloon endoscope is used, the small intestine often forms concentric circles because of its insertion characteristics. In this case, the small intestine forms circles around the fan supported by the mesentery (Fig. 10.1.5). Under these conditions, the side facing the center of the concentric circles is the mesenteric side. When the endoscope tip is moved toward the center of the circles under fluoroscopic guidance, the wall coming into the endoscopic view is the one on the mesenteric side. In Crohn's disease, ulcers are often found longitudinally on the mesenteric side, and Meckel's diverticulum is characteristically found on the side opposite to the mesentery.

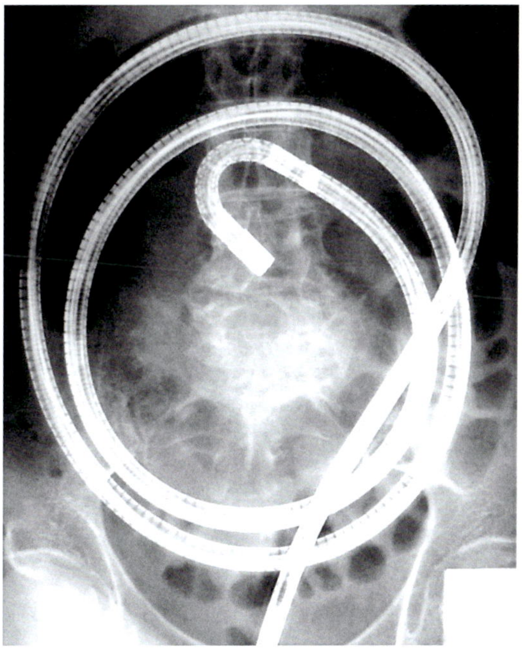

Fig. 10.1.5. Fluoroscopic image of a concentrically inserted endoscope

Double-balloon endoscope inserted through the anus

10.1.4 Selective Contrast-Enhanced Studies

Although a small bowel series is useful for obtaining objective images of lesions in the small intestine, it may be difficult to delineate lesions because some portions of the intestine intricately intertwine and overlap. Combining a contrast study and double-balloon endoscopy is useful because inflation of the balloon at the endoscope tip prevents backflow of a contrast agent and allows selective enhancement (Fig. 10.1.6).

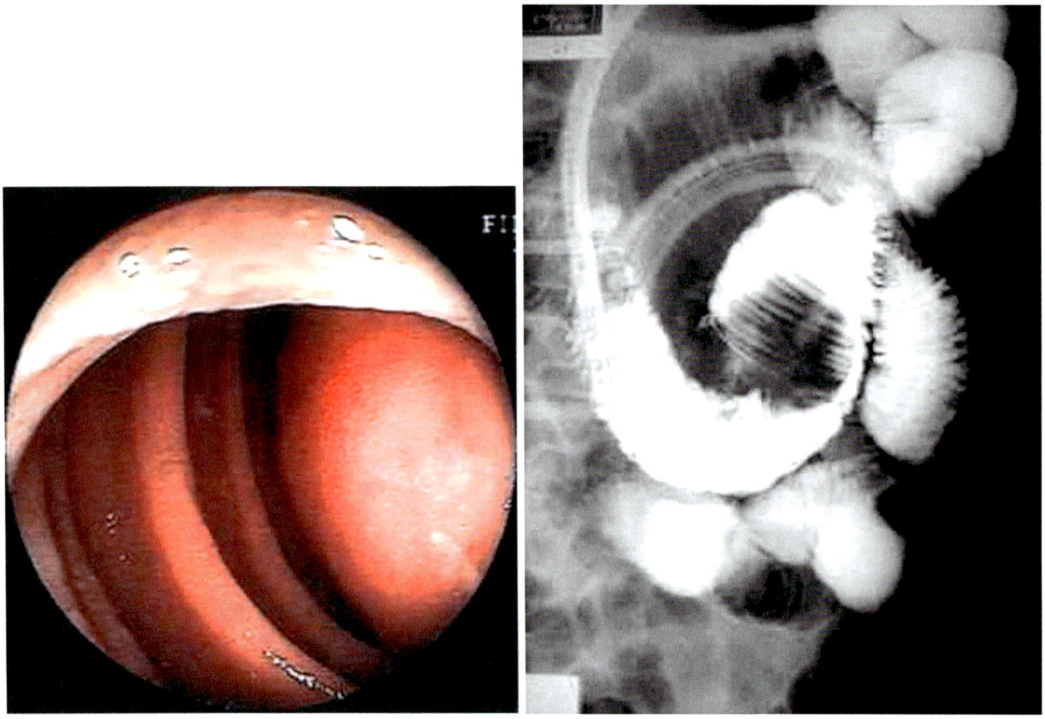

a b

Fig. 10.1.6. Endoscopic observation and selective, contrast-enhanced radiography with a double-balloon endoscope

a Endoscopic view of gastrointestinal stromal tumor (GIST) of the jejunum

b Selective, contrast-enhanced radiograph obtained with a double-balloon endoscope in the same patient

10.1.5 Other Studies

There seems to be other important information on endoscopic diagnosis in the small intestine. However, endoscopic observation of the distal small intestine has just started, and the accumulation of clinical experience is important.

10.2 Small-Intestinal Tumor

It was previously difficult to diagnose a small-intestinal tumor and to make a histological diagnosis of a radiographically suspected tumor unless exploratory laparotomy was performed. Double-balloon endoscopy is an epoch-making technique in that it allows insertion of the endoscope into the distal small intestine, endoscopic tissue biopsy, and aggressive endoscopic treatment of tumor bleeding. This subsection presents cases of small-intestinal tumors identified or treated by double-balloon endoscopy and those for which treatment strategies were determined by the modality, thereby demonstrating the diagnostic value and therapeutic potential of double-balloon endoscopy in small-intestinal tumors.

10.2.1 Small-Intestinal Tumor: Incidence

The incidence of small-intestinal tumors has been reported to account for 5% of primary gastrointestinal tumors [1], but the incidence appears to be much higher. To date, 74% of benign tumors are identified by pathological autopsy, and 75% of malignancies are found when symptoms develop [2]. Although a small-intestinal tumor is less symptomatic, intermittent abdominal pain, intestinal obstruction, and vomiting may occur regardless of whether the tumor is primary, metastatic, malignant, or benign. Signs include anemia, abdominal mass, and weight loss. It is important to take a small-intestinal tumor into consideration in patients 50 years of age or older who have fecal occult blood associated with iron deficiency anemia but no tumor of the large intestine [2]. Frequently reported benign tumors in the literature include adenoma, gastrointestinal stromal tumors (GISTs), lipoma, and hemangioma; and these four types of tumor account for 90% of the total. Malignancies of the small intestine account for 2% or less of all malignancies of the gastrointestinal tract. The malignancies occur most frequently in individuals in their fifties and twice as often in men as in women. The common histological types include adenocarcinoma, carcinoid, and lymphoma [3]. We have used a double-balloon endoscope to directly observe and diagnose GISTs, inflammatory fibroid polyps (IFP), adenocarcinoma, lymphoma, and metastatic large cell carcinoma.

10.2.2 Small-Intestinal Tumors Revealed by Double-Balloon Endoscopy

10.2.2.1 *Gastrointestinal Stromal Tumor*

The GIST is the most common mesenchymal tumor that develops in the gastrointestinal tract. Most tumors previously called leiomyoma, schwannoma, leiomyoblastoma, and leiomyosarcoma are classified into a single category of GIST on the basis of molecular, biological, or immunohistological characteristics [1]. We have diagnosed multiple cases of GIST of the small intestine by double-balloon endoscopy.

Figure 10.2.1 shows a case of GIST in which no abnormalities were found by upper or lower gastrointestinal endoscopy performed to investigate repeated melena. The diagnosis was made on the basis of biopsy specimens obtained by double-balloon endoscopy [4]. The endoscopy revealed a rather sharply protruding submucosal tumor with a bleeding ulcer on the top (Fig. 10.2.1a); a similar finding was shown by selective, contrast-enhanced radiography (Fig. 10.2.1b). After a histologically confirmed diagnosis, partial resection of the small intestine was performed (Fig. 10.2.1c).

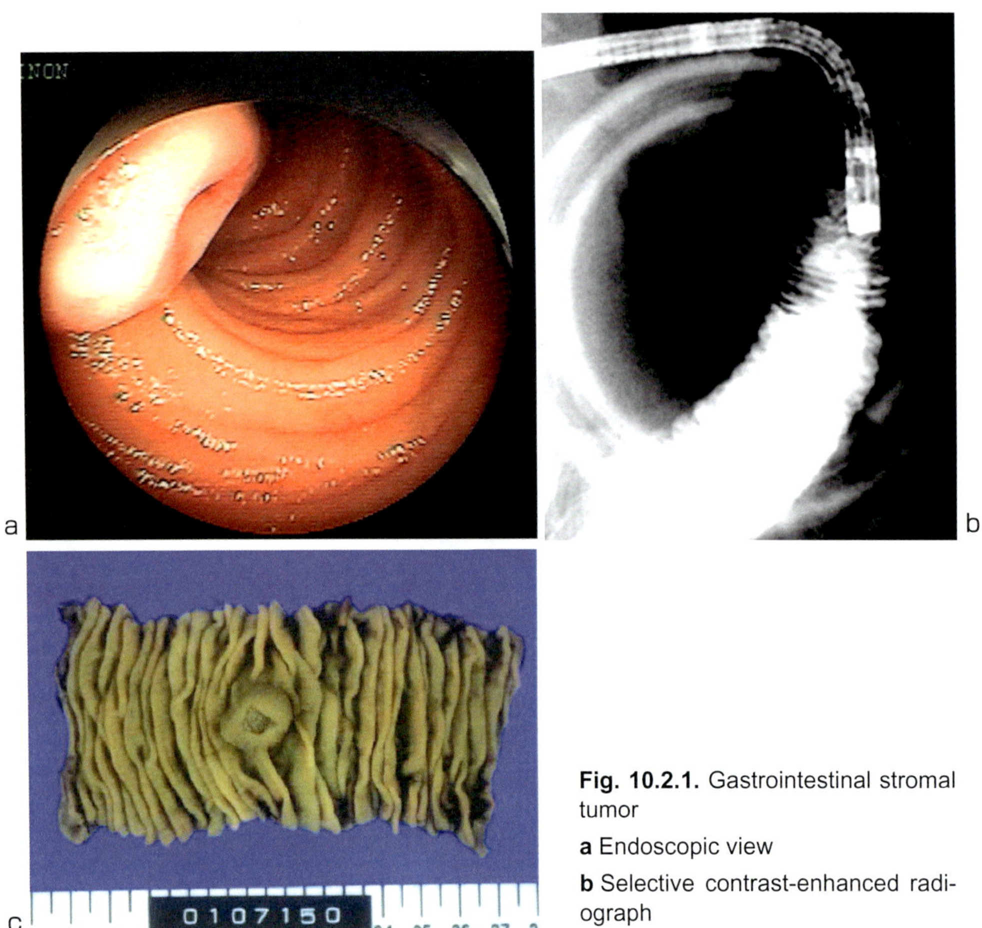

Fig. 10.2.1. Gastrointestinal stromal tumor

a Endoscopic view

b Selective contrast-enhanced radiograph

c Surgical specimen

10.2.2.2 *Inflammatory Fibroid Polyp*

The inflammatory fibroid polyp (IFP), characterized by proliferation of mesenchymal cells, most frequently occurs in individuals about 60 years of age; it most commonly involves the stomach followed by the large intestine and the small intestine. It is a benign lesion that develops in the submucosal layer. It occurs slightly more frequently in women. The tumor itself is asymptomatic and may be associated with symptoms of intussusception and melena [5]. Figure 10.2.2 shows a patient with lower abdominal pain in whom intussusception was suspected on abdominal radiography, followed by a diagnosis of intussusception associated with small-intestinal tumor by CT, a diagnosis of IFP on the basis of biopsy specimens obtained by double-balloon endoscopy, and surgical resection [6].

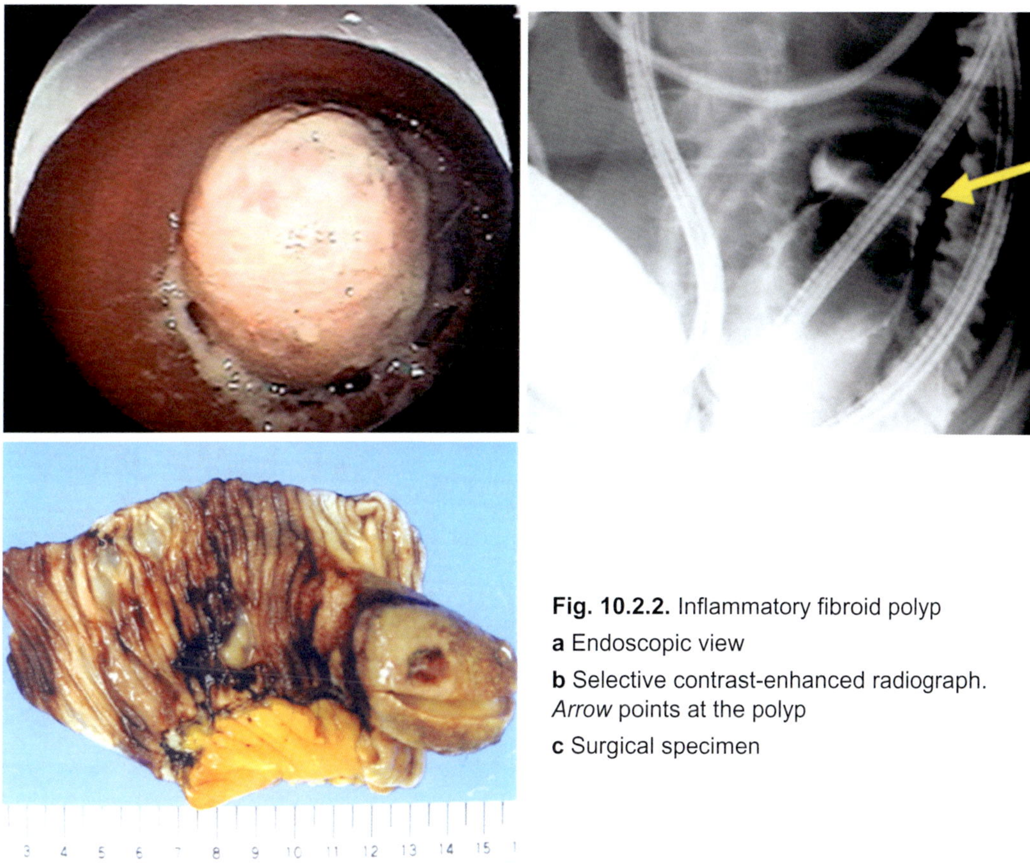

Fig. 10.2.2. Inflammatory fibroid polyp

a Endoscopic view

b Selective contrast-enhanced radiograph. *Arrow* points at the polyp

c Surgical specimen

10.2.2.3 Adenocarcinoma

Small intestinal adenocarcinoma accounts for 0.3% of all malignancies of the gastrointestinal tract and 30% to 50% of all malignancies of the small intestine [7]. Previously, most cases were subjected to surgery after symptoms such as obstruction and anemia developed; lymph node metastasis had already occurred when the cancer was found, indicating a poor prognosis. The 5-year survival rate is 15% to 30% [8]. Figure 10.2.3 shows a case of an epithelial tumor with an ulcer mound located 50 cm away from the ligament of Treitz. Double-balloon endoscopy was performed for a thorough examination of recurrent obstructive symptoms (Fig. 10.2.3a), and it revealed the tumor. A diagnosis of adenocarcinoma was made based on the endoscopic and selective contrast-enhanced radiography (Fig. 10.2.3b) findings and was confirmed by biopsy.

a 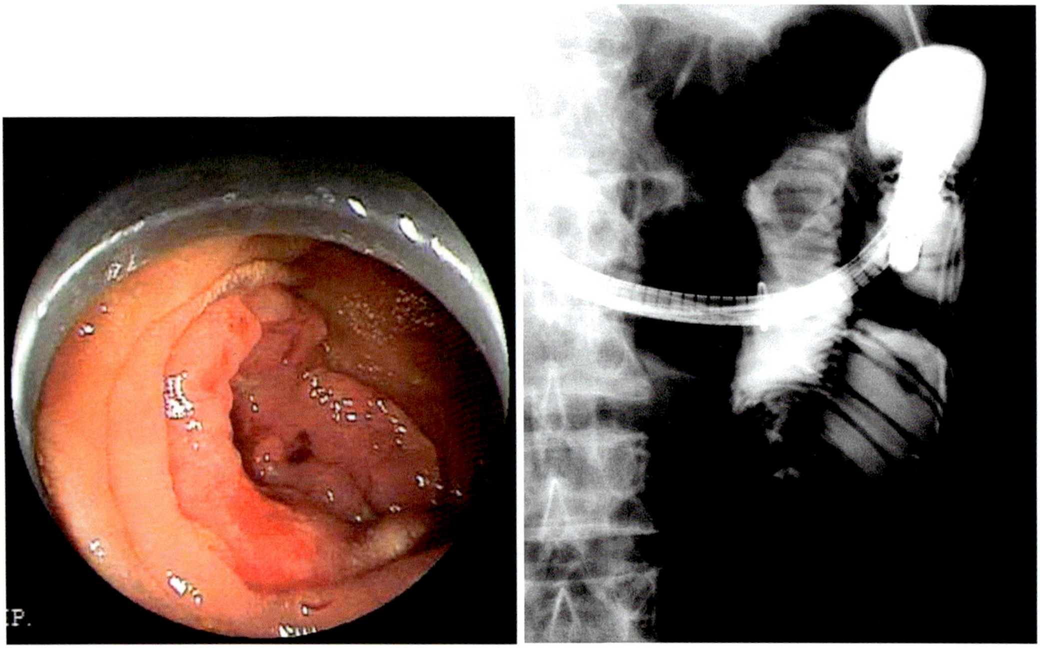 b

Fig. 10.2.3. Jejunal adenocarcinoma

a Endoscopic view

b Selective contrast-enhanced radiograph

10.2.2.4 *Malignant Lymphoma*

Malignant lymphoma of the gastrointestinal tract accounts for 5% to 20% of non-Hodgkin's B-cell lymphoma. The stomach is the most common site of occurrence, and the small intestine is also commonly involved. Like adenocarcinoma, most patients have advanced lymphoma at the time of diagnosis by conventional endoscopy, with a poor prognosis; the 5-year survival rate is approximately 25% [7].

The endoscopic view (Fig. 10.2.4a) and selective contrast-enhanced radiograph (Fig. 10.2.4b) show a case of malignant lymphoma diagnosed by double-balloon endoscopy. The procedure was performed because bleeding from the upper jejunum was suspected based on tarry stools and significant anemia with a hemoglobin level of 4.1 g/dl [9].

a

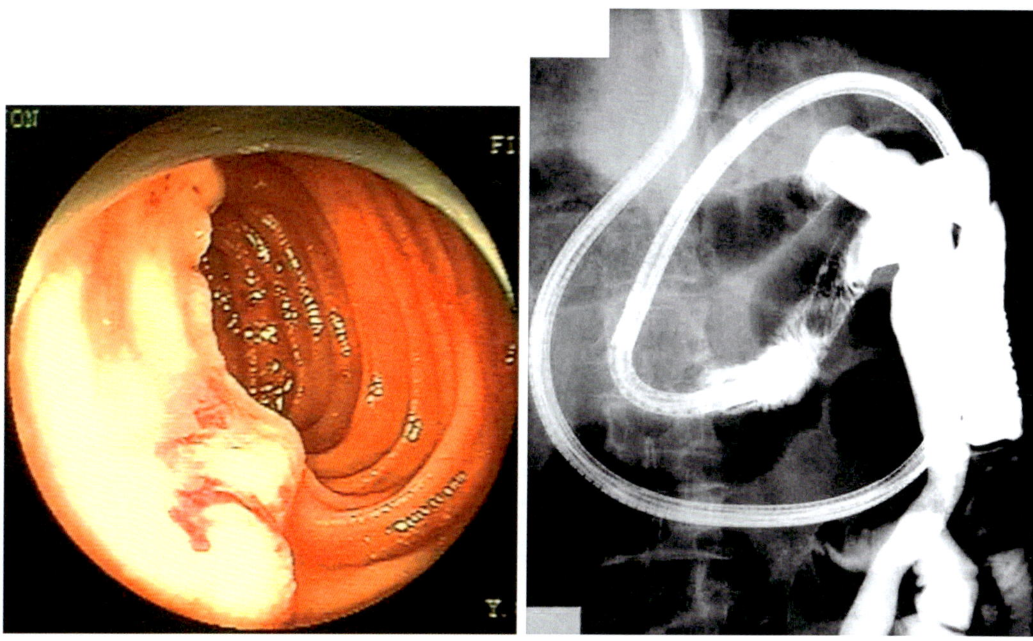

b

Fig. 10.2.4. Malignant lymphoma

a Endoscopic view

b Selective contrast-enhanced radiograph

10.2.2.5 *Metastatic Large Cell Carcinoma*

It has been reported that 9.7% of metastases of pulmonary large-cell carcinoma occur in the gastrointestinal tract and 5.7% in the small intestine, indicating that it is not an uncommon disorder [10]. Its symptoms include gastrointestinal bleeding with anemia. A patient who had undergone resection of a lung cancer a few years earlier underwent double-balloon endoscopy for a thorough examination of gastrointestinal bleeding (Fig. 10.2.5a). Contrast-enhanced radiography showed a mass (Fig. 10.2.5b). Biopsy resulted in a diagnosis of large-cell carcinoma, and the past history suggested metastasis of lung cancer. Partial resection of the small intestine was performed (Fig. 10.2.5c).

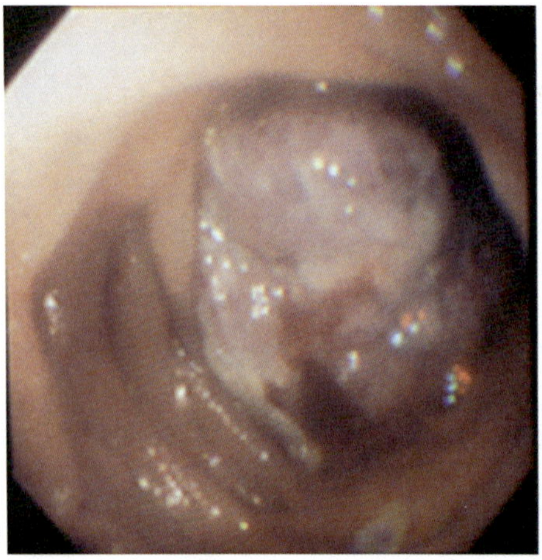
a

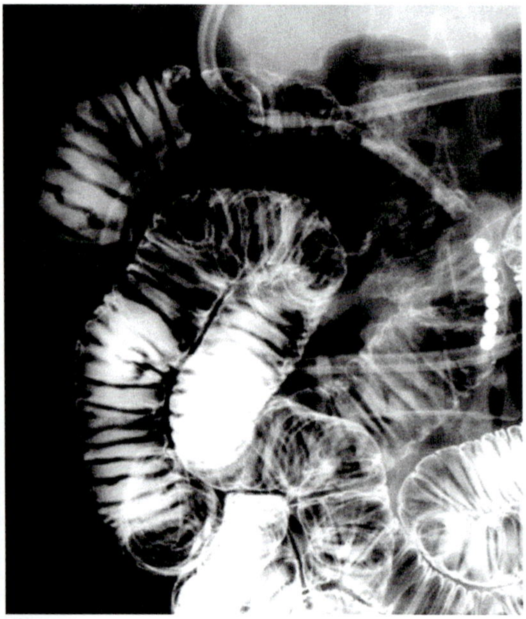
b

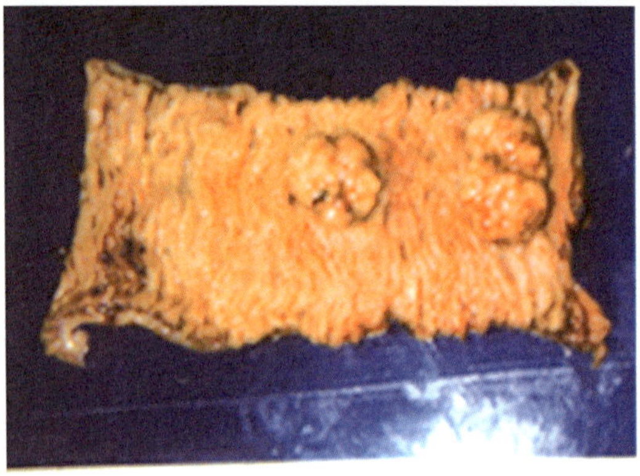
c

Fig. 10.2.5. Metastatic large cell carcinoma

a Endoscopic view

b Contrast-enhanced radiograph

c Surgical specimenograph

References

1. Hirota S, Isozaki K, Moriyama Y, et al (1998) Gain-of-function of c-kit in human gastrointestinal stromal tumors. Science 279:577–580
2. Rossini FP, Risio M (1998) Small bowel tumors. In: Rossini FP, Gay G (eds) Atlas of Enteroscopy. Springer, Milan, pp 125–135
3. Ojha A, Zacherl J, Scheuba C, et al (2000) Primary small bowel malignancies: single center results of three decades. J Clin Gastroenterol 30:289–293
4. Nishimura M, Yamamoto H, Kita H, et al (2004) A case of gastrointestinal stromal tumor in the jejunum: diagnosis and control of bleeding with electrocoagulation by using double-balloon enteroscopy. J Gastroenterol 39:1001–1004
5. Ozolek JA, Sasatomi E, Swalsky PA, et al (2004) Inflammatory fibroid polyps of the gastrointestinal tract: clinical, pathologic, and molecular characteristics. Appl Immunohistochem Mol Morphol 12:59–66
6. Miyata T, Yamamoto H, Kita H, et al (2004) A case of inflammatory fibroid polyp causing small bowel intussusception in which retrograde double-balloon enteroscopy was useful for the preoperative diagnosis. Endoscopy 36:344–347
7. Maglint DDT, Herlinger H, Birnbaum BA (eds) (1999) Clinical imaging of the small intestine, 2nd ed. Springer, New York, pp 377–438
8. Satinder SG, Douglas MH, Anastasios AM (2001) Small intestinal neoplasms. J Clin Gastroenterol 33:267–282
9. Hashimoto A, Yamamoto H, Yano T, et al (2003) Successful hemostasis of bleeding malignant lymphoma with a enteroscope by double-balloon method. Prog Dig Endosc 62:104–105
10. Ryo H, Sakai H, Ikeda T, et al (1996) Gastrointestinal metastasis from lung cancer. Nihon Kyobu Shikkan Gakkai Zasshi 34:968–972

10.3 Stenosis of the Small Intestine

10.3.1 Stenosis of the Small Intestine: Description

Endoscopic investigation of stenotic lesions, as well as bleeding in the small intestine, is an indication for which the double-balloon endoscope offers the greatest advantage. Stenosis of the small intestine often interferes with the passage of intestinal contents and thereby causes bowel obstruction symptoms, such as abdominal pain, abdominal distension, and vomiting. Particularly in the distal small intestine, however, stenosis is less symptomatic unless severe narrowing occurs because intestinal contents are usually well-digested liquids. It is difficult to delineate stenosis of the small intestine by modalities other than contrast-enhanced studies, and the diagnosis is difficult to make particularly when symptoms chronically persist. Consequently, patients often suffer from symptoms due to stenosis of the small intestine for a long time. Accurate diagnosis of the cause of stenosis of the small intestine and selection of appropriate treatment often relieve years of distress and afford great satisfaction to patients.

10.3.2 Bowel Obstruction of the Small Intestine

Bowel obstruction of the small intestine is a common disease in daily clinical practice. In patients with previous surgery, bowel obstruction of the small intestine is most likely to result from postoperative intestinal adhesion. When stenosis of the small intestine is suspected on the basis of bowel obstruction symptoms, however, a thorough examination is needed to identify the cause of the stenosis because stenosis of the small intestine is caused by not only adhesions but also a variety of conditions, such as ischemia, ulcer, and tumor. Patients with suspected stenosis of the small intestine are often admitted to hospital for bowel obstruction symptoms. In principle, intestinal rest and conservative therapy are provided to improve the condition of the patients. In principle, contrast-enhanced studies, computed tomography (CT), magnetic resonance imaging (MRI), conventional upper endoscopy, or lower endoscopy should be performed after the bowel obstruction conditions have resolved, and enteroscopy may be considered. In some patients, after decompression with a long decompression tube, a balloon-attached overtube may be inserted with a long decompression tube as a guide, which facilitates insertion of an endoscope to the region that the tip of a long decompression tube has reached (see a long decompression tube guiding method in section 12.2).

10.3.3 Diagnosis of Stenosis of the Small Intestine

A variety of diseases may cause stenosis of the small intestine (Table 10.3.1), and it is essential to make an accurate diagnosis in patients with stenotic lesions. Diagnosis requires inserting an endoscope to the stenotic site. Like double-balloon endoscopy, capsule endoscopy is an epoch-making method that allows total enteroscopy. However, capsule endoscopy should not be performed to observe stenotic lesions because of the risk of retaining the capsule. Double-balloon endoscopy is superior to capsule endoscopy in that it can be performed through the mouth and the anus and that stenosis is not a contraindication to this method. When the examination is performed through the anus, however, preparation with polyethylene glycol electrolyte solution may involve risk depending on the degree of stenosis (see Chapter 6). In this case, the examination must be performed with minimum preparation by high enema to cleanse the large intestine. Regardless of the oral or anal approach, unnecessary air insufflation is avoided during insertion, and care is taken not to place strain on the stenotic site of the intestine.

10.3.4 Double-Balloon Endoscopy for Stenosis of the Small Intestine

Before enteroscopy, evaluation of clinical symptoms, plain abdominal radiography, CT, MRI, or a contrast-enhanced study should be performed to estimate whether the jejunum or the ileum is involved. The location where the internal diameter of the intestine dramatically changes should be explored; however, examination of the entire small intestine is often required because of uncertainty about the stenotic site. In those cases, the endoscope should be inserted through the anus and the remaining region examined through the mouth.

First, the endoscope is advanced to the stenotic site to observe the lesions. When epithelial changes protruding into the lumen due to a tumor or inflammation are found, the differential diagnosis of lesions can be made by routine observation. In most cases, histological examination leads to definite diagnosis. When no gross change in the luminal epithelium is found in the stenosis of the small intestine, adhesion, intestinal ischemia, nonepithelial tumor, and extrinsic compression by tumor outside the intestine should be considered. When a severe stenosis makes it difficult to direct endoscopic observation of the stenotic lumen, a selective contrast-enhanced study with the balloons of the endoscope and the overtube inflated before the stenotic site allows evaluation of the degree and length of the stenosis and provides useful information for the diagnosis. After contrast enhancement, a biopsy forceps may be carefully inserted under fluoroscopic guidance to collect tissues. In cases of inflammatory stenosis associated with ulcerative lesions, such as tuberculosis and Crohn's disease, particularly with new ulcers, careful judgment is required when the endoscope or the overtube is inserted beyond the stenotic site even if the stenosis allows passage of the endoscope because the passage of the endoscope or the overtube and balloon inflation may cause perforation by applying pressure to the affected area. In the presence of these ulcerative lesions, tissue sampling from the ulcer base should be avoided to prevent perforation.

Stenosis of the small intestine often occurs as a single lesion but may occur as multiple lesions, as in Crohn's disease. When the endoscope reveals a stenotic lesion in the small intestine and fails to pass through the lesion, a selective contrast-enhanced study with balloon inflation, as described above, is useful for obtaining information on the distal end of the stenotic site. Tattooing in the vicinity of the stenotic site requiring treatment is useful for identifying the lesion from the serosal side during surgery when laparoscopic treatment is required later.

Table 10.3.1. Diseases that may cause stenosis of the small intestine

Benign inflammatory stenosis
Crohn's disease
NSAID-induced ulcer
Behçet's disease
Intestinal tuberculosis
Nonspecific multiple ulcers of the small intestine
Traumatic ischemic stenosis of the small intestine
Anticoagulant bowel obstruction
Small-intestinal tumor
Postoperative intestinal adhesion
Stenosis of the small intestine after pancreatitis
Compression by lesions outside of the intestine

10.3.5 Endoscopic Treatment of Stenosis of the Small Intestine

Stenosis of the small intestine found by endoscopy requires determining a treatment strategy. For stenosis associated with benign disease, it should be determined in principle whether the stenosis can be treated by endoscopic dilatation (see section 11.4). Although endoscopic dilatation of stenosis of the small intestine is believed to be an important procedure that will develop further, the risk of dilatation-related perforation should always be taken into consideration. For the establishment of indications for endoscopic dilatation, it should be determined which lesions can be treated safely by dilatation and whether dilatation is expected to provide long-term alleviation of clinical symptoms on the basis of accumulated clinical data. For stenosis of the small intestine associated with malignant disease, resection of the affected intestine is considered after the curability of the lesion is determined by whole-body screening. In some cases, however, intervention is limited to bypass surgery alone. Endoscopic stenting may be considered when long-term survival is unlikely, surgery under general anesthesia is difficult because of underlying disease, or patients refuse to undergo surgery (see section 11.4).

● Case 1

Images of stenosis in bowel obstruction of the small intestine caused by submucosal hematoma in a patient receiving an anticoagulant (anticoagulant bowel obstruction) (Fig. 10.3.1) [1].

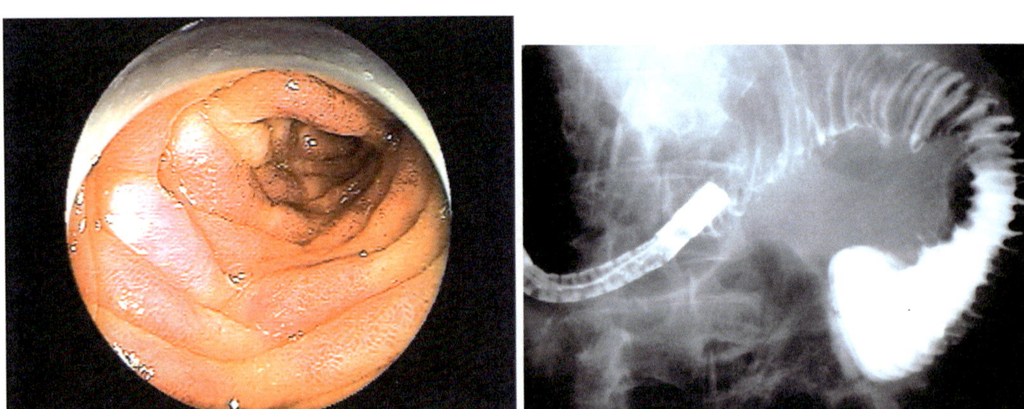

a b

Fig. 10.3.1. Anticoagulant bowel obstruction

a Endoscopic view

b Selective contrast-enhanced radiograph

● Case 2

Endoscopic dilatation of stenosis of the small intestine in a patient with Crohn's disease (Fig. 10.3.2) [2].

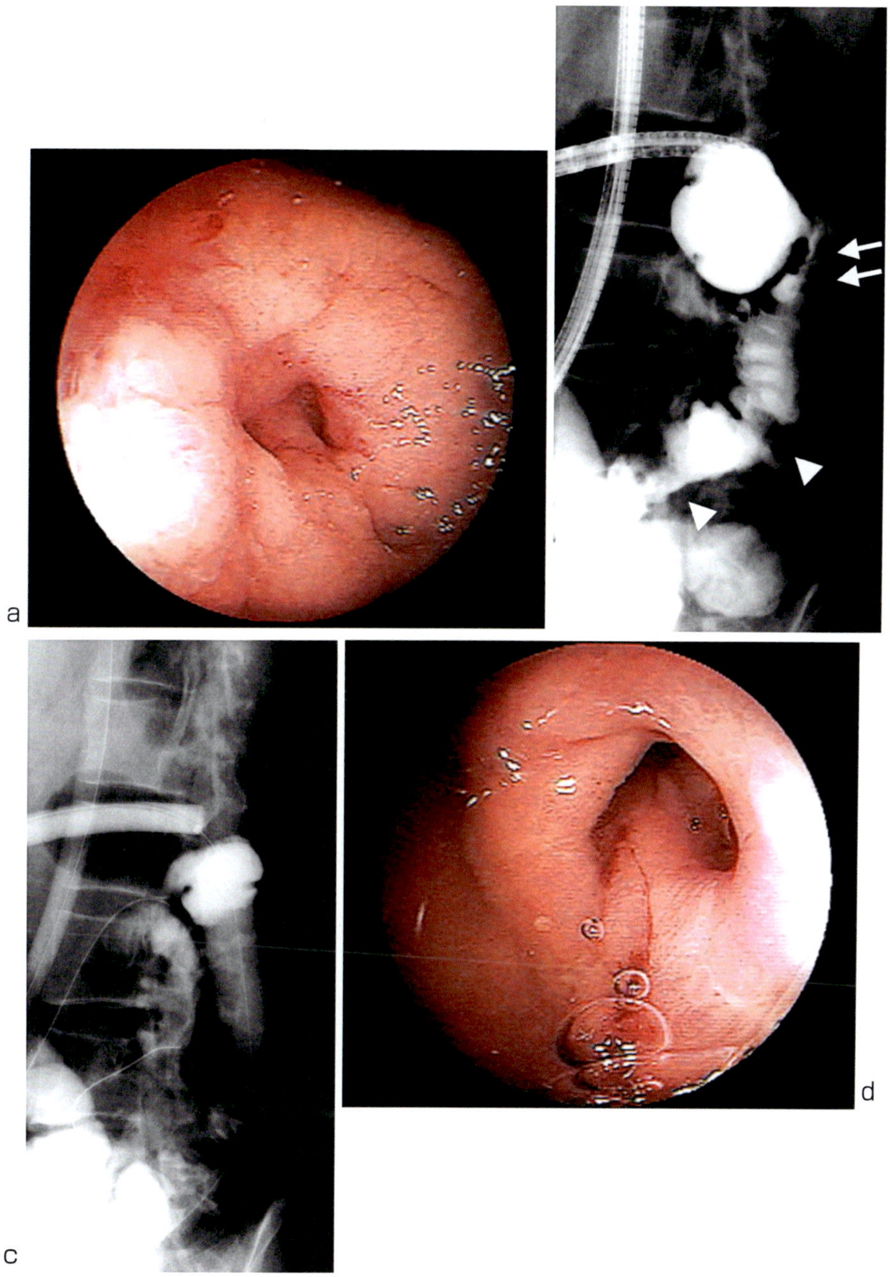

Fig. 10.3.2. Jejunal stenosis due to Crohn's disease

a Endoscopic view

b Contrast-enhanced radiograph of stenosis before dilatation

c Dilatation of stenosis with a balloon dilator inserted under fluoroscopic guidance after guidewire placement and endoscope removal. Arrows indicate strictures before dilatation; arrowheads indicate additional strictures at the distal site.

d Endoscopic view after dilatation

References

1. Shinozaki S, Yamamoto H, Kita H, et al (2004) Case report: direct observation with double-balloon enteroscopy of an intestinal intramural hematoma resulting in anticoagulant ileus. Dig Dis Sci 49:902–905
2. Sunada K, Yamamoto H, Kita H, et al (2004) Case report: successful treatment with balloon dilatation in combination with double-balloon enteroscopy of a stricture in the small bowel of a patient with Crohn's disease. Dig Endosc 16:237–240

10.4 Intestinal Ulcers and Erosions

Previously, the small intestine was believed to be an organ with few lesions. However, double-balloon endoscopy has revealed a variety of lesions. This subsection focuses on endoscopic views of ulcerative and erosive lesions in the small intestine.

10.4.1 Crohn's Disease

Crohn's disease consists of granulomatous inflammatory lesions with edema and ulcers and may occur in any part of the gastrointestinal tract from the mouth to the anus. In the small intestine, the ileum is preferentially affected. Endoscopic findings include a variety of ulcers, such as discontinuous or regional cobblestone appearance, longitudinal ulcers, aphthoid ulcers, and irregular ulcers. In patients with long-standing disease, repeated fibrosis may result in intestinal stenosis. Histologically, formation of noncaseating epithelioid cell granulomas is characteristic (Fig. 10.4.1).

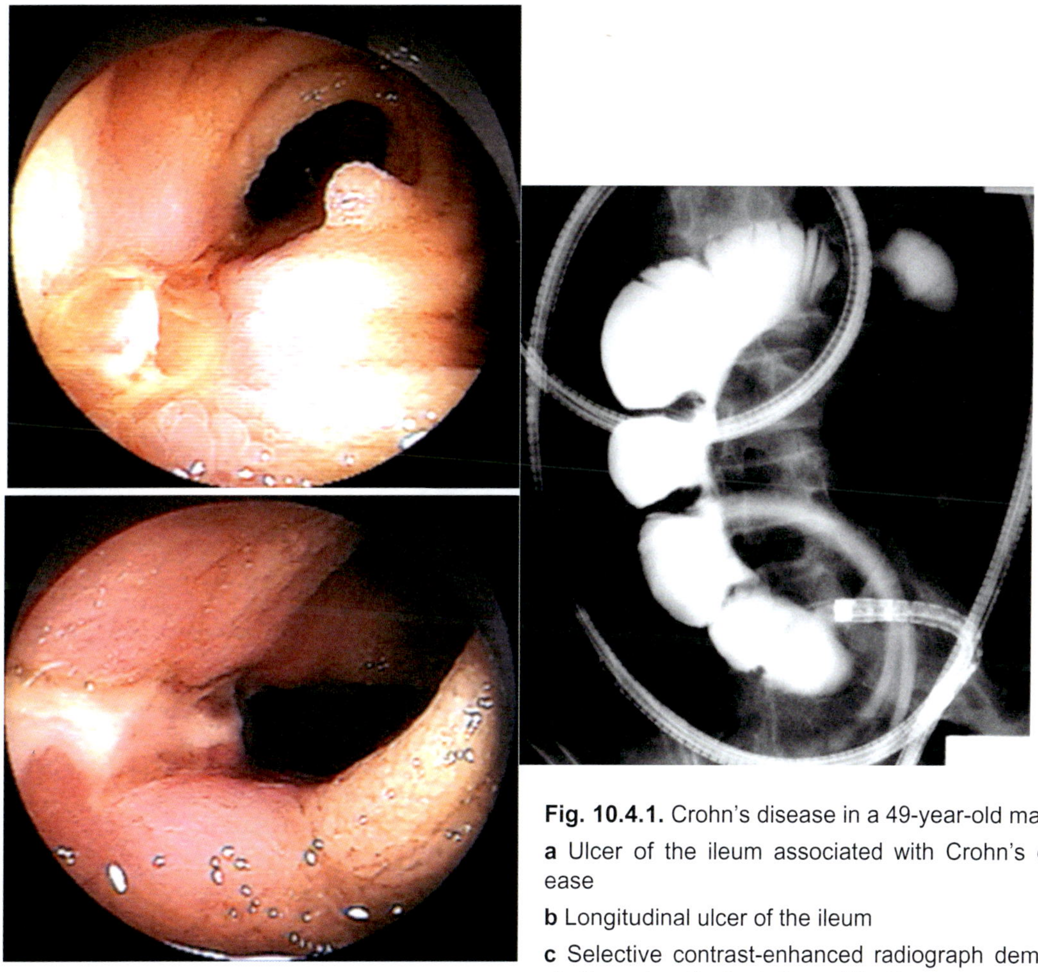

a

b

c

Fig. 10.4.1. Crohn's disease in a 49-year-old man

a Ulcer of the ileum associated with Crohn's disease

b Longitudinal ulcer of the ileum

c Selective contrast-enhanced radiograph demonstrating a longitudinal ulcer of the ileum

10.4.2 Intestinal Behçet's Disease

Behçet's disease is a systemic inflammatory disease of unknown etiology with primary symptoms of recurrent oral aphtha, skin symptoms, eye symptoms, and vulval ulcers. The disease, accompanied by intestinal lesions, is called intestinal Behçet's disease. Common intestinal lesions include round or oval deep ulcers in the ileocecal region. In some cases, however, ulcerative lesions are not present in the ileocecal region but are present in other regions in the small intestine; therefore, examination of the distal small intestine by double-balloon endoscopy is useful. There may be atypical lesions, such as small, shallow ulcers and aphthoid ulcers in the large intestine. Histological findings of the lesions are nonspecific chronic inflammatory changes without specific characteristics (Fig. 10.4.2).

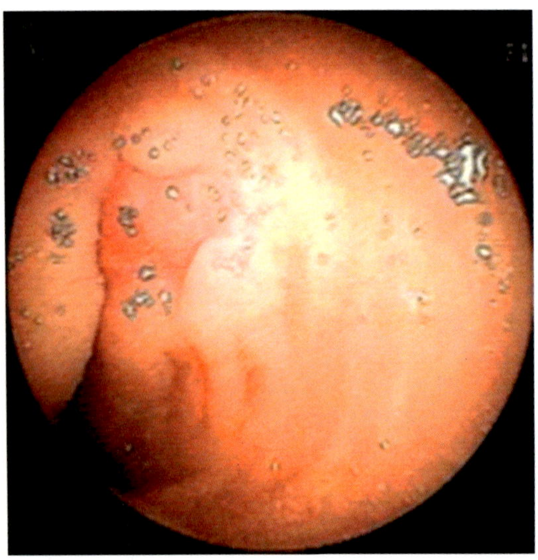

Fig. 10.4.2. Deep ulcer in the middle of the ileum of a 65-year-old woman with Behçet's disease

In this case, no lesion was found in the ileocecal region

Advice

Ulcerative Lesion and Surrounding Villi

Swollen or edematous villi are often found around ulcerative lesions in the small intestine. When the double-balloon endoscope is used to observe the small intestine, attention should be given to villous abnormalities in the field of view to locate ulcerative lesions. These appear to be a consequence of the influence of inflammation of localized lesions on the surrounding villi.

10.4.3 NSAID-Induced, Small-Intestinal Ulcer

Allison et al. reported that autopsies revealed small-intestinal ulcers in 8.4% of patients receiving nonsteroidal antiinflammatory drugs (NSAIDs) for a long time [1]. In daily clinical practice, patients who are prescribed NSAIDs for relief of pain associated with rheumatic disease or arthropathy often have manifestations of melena and anemia of unknown cause. Many of these lesions are not accompanied by ulcers of the stomach, duodenum, large intestine, or terminal ileum that are accessible by upper or lower gastrointestinal endoscopy, and it is one of the diseases for which endoscopic diagnosis was previously difficult to make. However, examination of the entire small intestine with the double-balloon endoscope now allows diagnosis and localization of ulcers of the distal small intestine. Kessler et al. reported that lesions were found more frequently in the ileum than in the jejunum in patients with previous surgeries [2]. A variety of changes were found by endoscopy, including deep round ulcers, annular ulcers, and erosions; and diaphragmatic strictures were found in some patients who had been taking NSAIDs for a long time [3,4]. Histological examination shows nonspecific ulcers. In general, symptoms of melena and anemia diminish soon after discontinuation of oral NSAIDs (Fig. 10.4.3) [5].

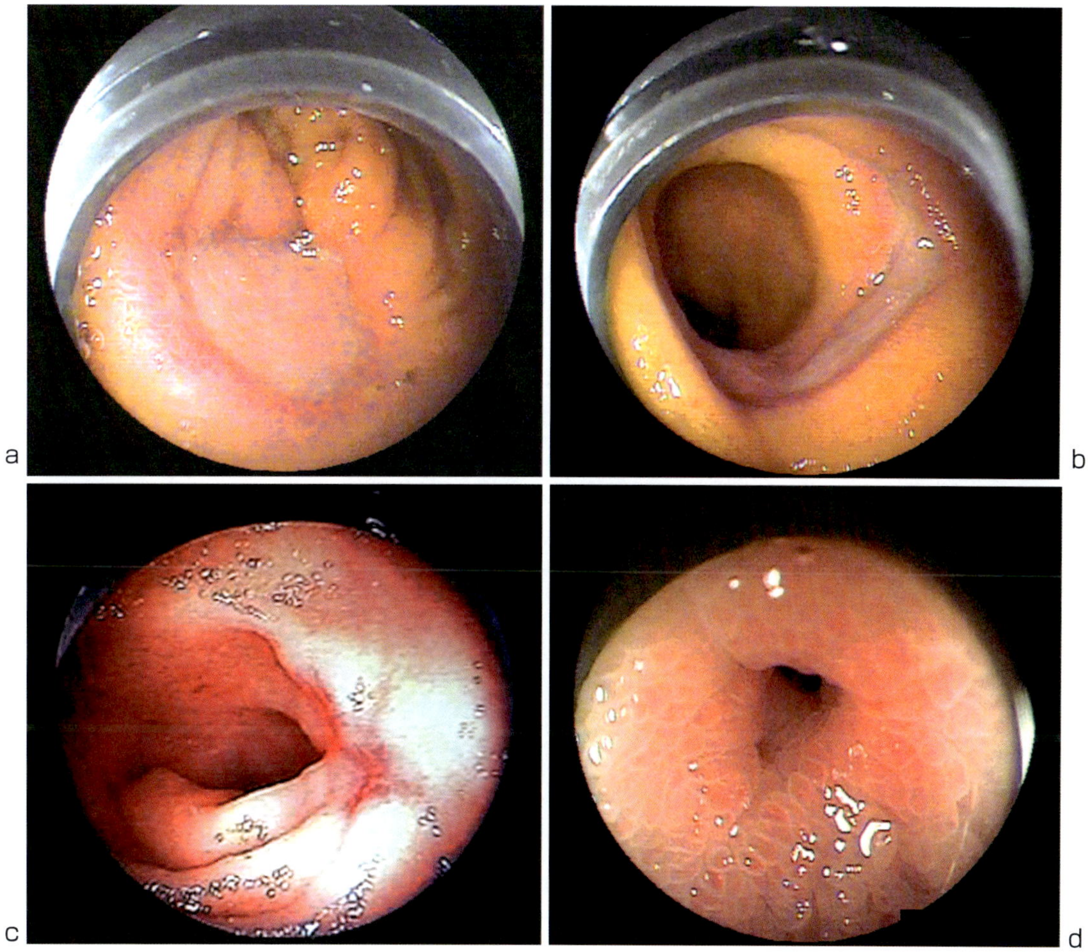

Fig. 10.4.3. NSAID-induced small-intestinal ulcer

a NSAID-induced ileal ulcer in a 67-year-old woman receiving oral diclofenac sodium

b Annular ulcer of the ileum in the patient in **a**

c NSAID-induced bleeding ulcer of the ileum in a 76-year-old woman taking oral diclofenac sodium

d Circumferential stenosis of the ileum in a patient who had been taking oral NSAIDs for a long time

10.4.4 Meckel's Ulcer

Meckel's diverticulum results from postnatal incomplete obliteration of the omphalomesenteric duct adjacent to the intestine. In adults, it is located in the ileum 30–100 cm from the ileocecal valve and on the side opposite to the mesentery. A diverticular intestine on the mesenteric side is likely to be intestinal duplication (see "Advice, Intestinal duplication," below). Gastric acid secreted from the fundic gland of the ectopic gastric mucosa in the diverticulum may cause ulcers of the diverticulum or the ileal mucosa in the vicinity of the diverticulum, leading to abdominal pain, gastrointestinal bleeding, or gastrointestinal perforation. It may also cause intestinal obstruction, intussusception, or diverticulitis (Fig. 10.4.4).

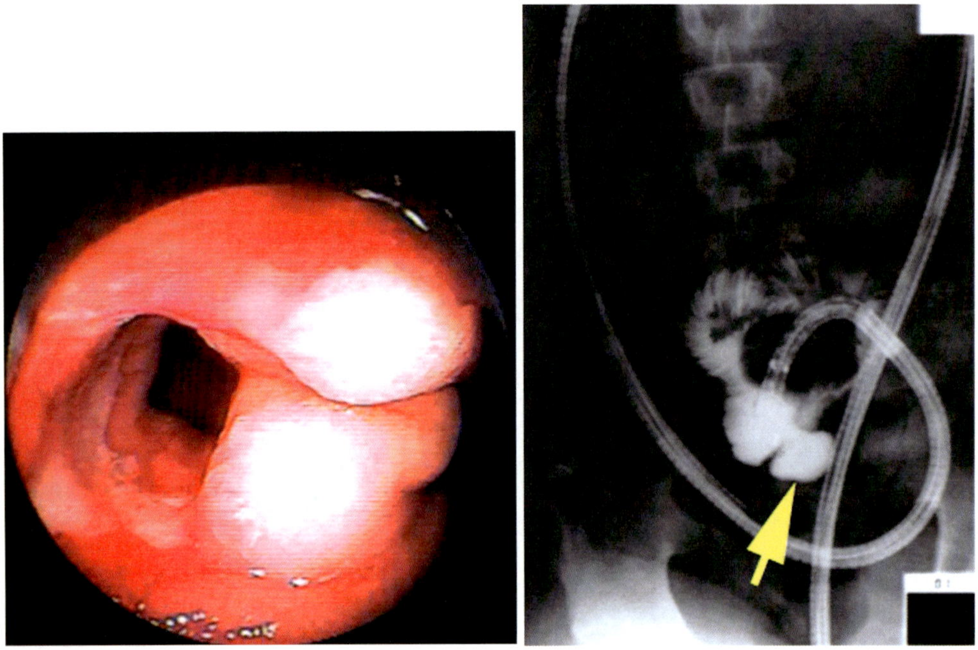

a b

Fig. 10.4.4. Meckel's diverticulum in a 19-year-old man

a Meckel's diverticulum with an ulcer of its opening in the ileum

b Selective, contrast-enhanced radiograph. Meckel's diverticulum is enhanced at the *arrow*

Advice

Intestinal Duplication

Intestinal duplication may occur in any region of the gastrointestinal tract, and there are many theories to explain the occurrence. The small intestine and the ileocecal region are often involved. Ectopic gastric mucosa may be found. In clinical practice, this condition often manifests as an intestinal obstruction due to direct compression of the adjacent intestine or intussusception with intestinal duplication as a lead point.

10.4.5 Multiple Hemorrhagic Erosions

Unexplained bleeding may be found due to multiple erosions of the small intestine. A patient was found to have multiple ileal erosions and minimal bleeding, for which endoscopic coagulation and hemostasis were performed (Fig. 10.4.5).

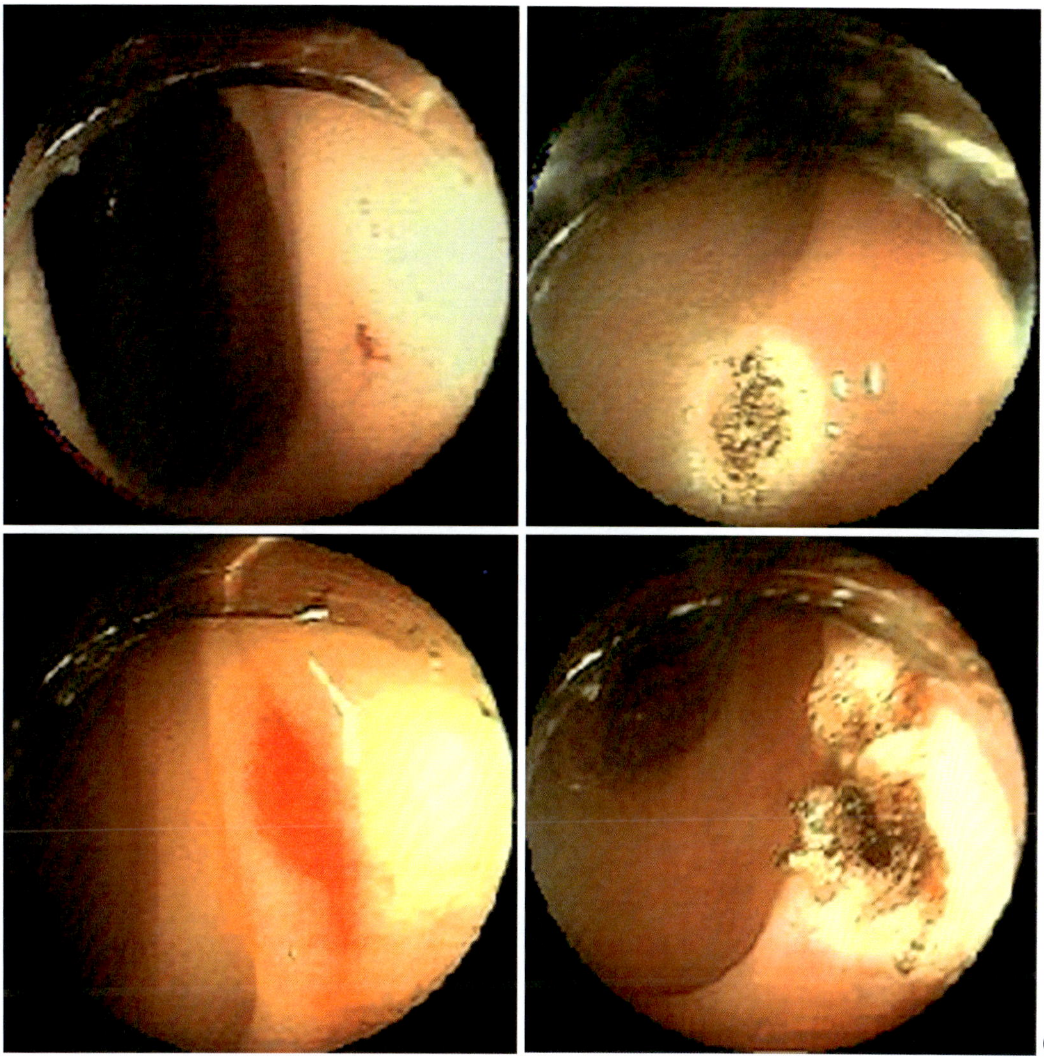

a b c d

Fig. 10.4.5. Multiple hemorrhagic erosions

a Mucosal erosion with bleeding in the ileum

b Coagulation and hemostasis were performed on the lesion in **a**

c Similar lesion at a different location of the ileum

d Similar treatment was performed on the lesion in **c**

Advice

On the Mesenteric Side or the Opposite Side?

Double-balloon endoscopy allows differentiation of lesions on the mesenteric side and those on the opposite side. The double-balloon endoscopy is inserted so it stretches the mesentery in a fan shape and forms concentric circles with the pivot as a center. The intestinal wall facing the center of concentric circles is on the mesenteric side. When the endoscope tip is moved toward the center of the circles under fluoroscopic guidance, the wall coming into the endoscopic view is the one on the mesenteric side.

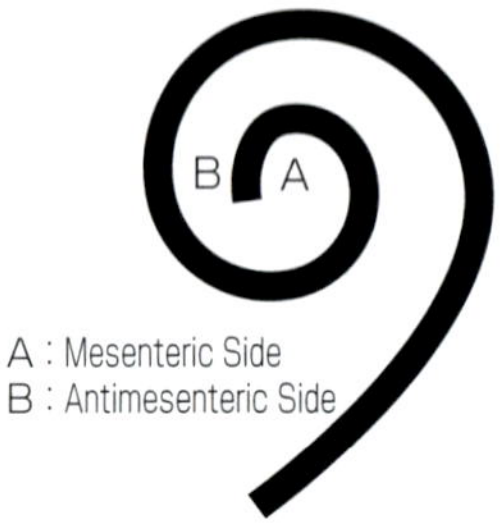

References

1. Allison MC, Howatson AG, Torrance CJ, et al (1992) Gastrointestinal damage associated with the use of nonsteroidal anti-inflammatory drugs. N Engl J Med 327:749–754
2. Kessler WF, Shires GT 3rd, Fahey TJ 3rd (1997) Surgical complications of nonsteroidal antiinflammatory drug-induced small bowel ulceration. J Am Coll Surg 185:250–254
3. Bjarnason I, Price AB, Zanelli G, et al (1988) Clinicopathological features of nonsteroidal anti-inflammatory drug-induced small intestinal strictures. Gastroenterology 94:1070–1074
4. Matsuhashi N, Yamada A, Hiraishi M, et al (1992) Multiple stricture of the small intestine after long-term nonsteroidal anti-inflammatory drug therapy. Am J Gastroenterol 87:1183–1186
5. Hayashi Y, Yamamoto H, Kita H, et al (2005) Non-steroidal anti-inflammatory drug-induced small bowel injuries identified by double-balloon endoscopy. World J Gastroenterol 11:4861–4864

10.5 Postoperative Intestinal Lesions

Except for Billroth I and II reconstructive operations, surgically anastomosed intestine is rarely accessible to endoscopy. Because double-balloon endoscopy allows support of any portion of the intestine and advancement of the endoscope in any direction, it enables observation of the afferent loop after Roux-en-Y anastomosis through which food does not pass and permits insertion against peristalsis. It allows observation of the bypassed and nonbypassed intestinal tracts as needed. In contrast, the antiperistaltic afferent loop and bypassed intestinal tracts cannot be observed with a capsule endoscope because it is not manipulable. Double-balloon endoscopy facilitates observation of the intestine that is otherwise inaccessible, which is expected to elucidate previously unknown pathological conditions in the postoperative intestine.

This subsection describes our experience: a case of multiple ulcers associated with blind loop syndrome occurring in the afferent loop after Roux-en-Y reconstruction and a case of adhesive intestinal obstruction in which the adhesion between the small intestine and the abdominal wall was successfully identified.

10.5.1 Blind Loop Syndrome

The blind loop syndrome, one of the malabsorption syndromes, is a collective name for pathological conditions manifesting as diarrhea, dyspepsia, malabsorption, and anemia that are caused by abnormal growth of intestinal bacterial flora associated with abnormal retention of intestinal contents in the intestinal tract [1]. Evidence suggests that the anemia in this syndrome is due to vitamin B_{12} deficiency, which may be caused by the use of vitamin B_{12} by intestinal bacteria and the binding of intestinal bacteria to the intrinsic factor–vitamin B_{12} complex.

● Case 1

A woman underwent cholecystectomy, choledochojejunostomy, and subtotal gastrectomy for organ damage due to a traffic accident at the age of 33 years. She began to have intermittent melena at age 40 years and was assigned a diagnosis of severe anemia. For investigation of the source of bleeding, she was admitted to our hospital and underwent double-balloon endoscopy at age 42. A long duodenal afferent loop was anastomosed to the jejunum by means of a Roux-en-Y anastomosis. Slightly longitudinal multiple ulcers were found in the afferent loop (Fig. 10.5.1a,b). Some of the ulcers were associated with oozing bleeding. These ulcers were found throughout the long afferent loop. Abnormal growth of intestinal bacterial flora in the blind loop was believed to be involved in the ulceration, and metronidazole (Flagyl) was given. Double-balloon endoscopy after 1 month of treatment showed an improvement in the ulcers with many scars (Fig. 10.5.1c,d). The primary cause of her anemia appeared to be chronic bleeding from multiple ulcers in the blind loop. This case suggests that potential multiple ulcers should be taken into consideration as a cause of anemia in patients with blind loop syndrome.

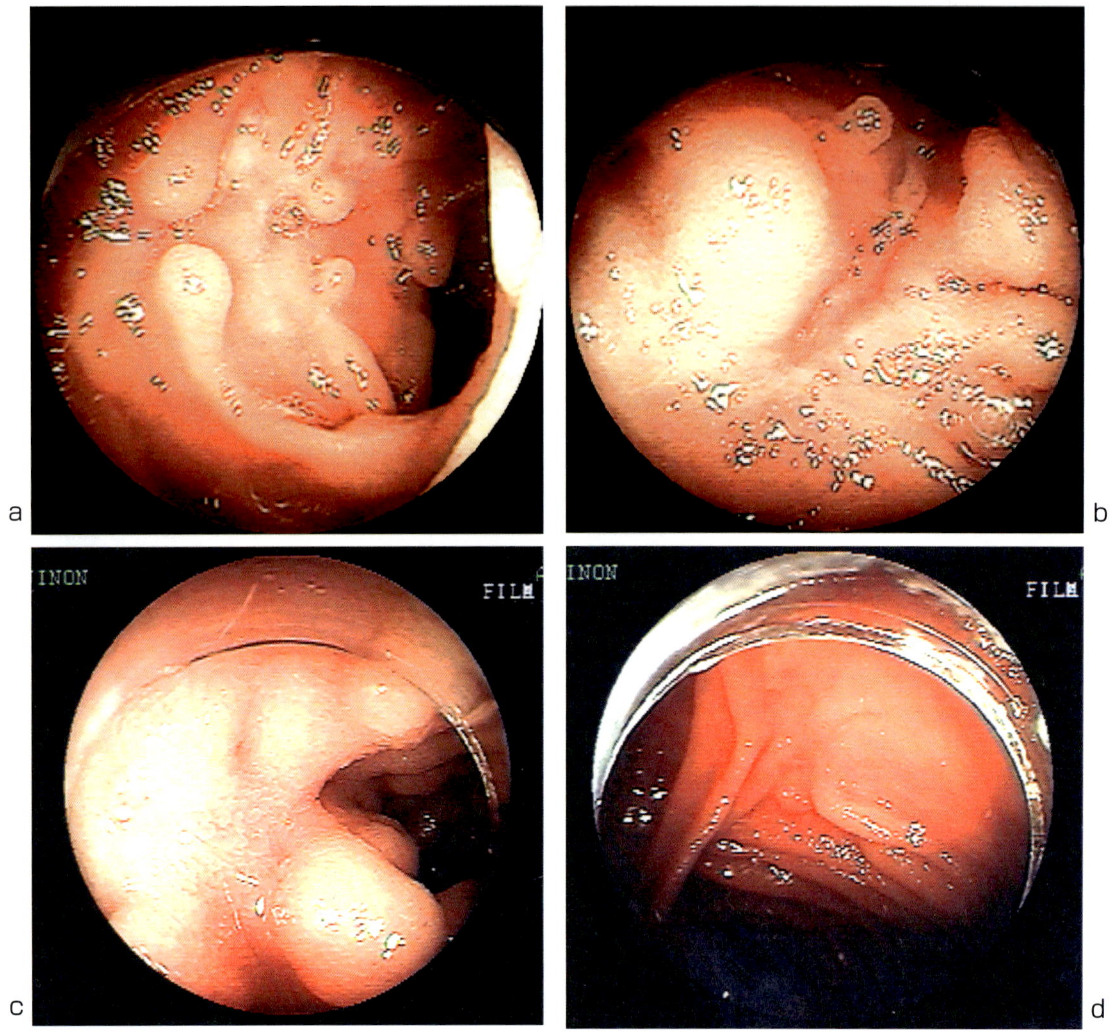

Fig. 10.5.1. Case 1. Blind loop syndrome

a Ulcer in the blind loop

b Longitudinal ulcer in the blind loop

c Ulcer scar after treatment with oral metronidazole

d Ulcer scar after treatment with oral metronidazole

10.5.2 Postoperative Adhesive Intestinal Obstructions

Adhesive intestinal obstructions are a common pathological condition after surgery. Unlike strangulation bowel obstruction accompanying circulatory disturbance, adhesive intestinal obstructions often improve with conservative treatment such as fasting and fluid therapy. However, it recurs in many patients, and thus saline cathartics and Chinese herbal medicines are given prophylactically. In patients with recurrent adhesive intestinal obstructions, identifying the adhesions and dividing them with minimally invasive laparoscopic surgery may be useful for improving the quality of life.

● Case 2

A 78-year-old man was admitted to our hospital for a thorough examination. At the age of 50 years, he had undergone emergency surgery for a rupture of the intestine and pelvic fracture due to an accident. The intestine was completely ruptured 150 cm from the terminal ileum, and end-to-end anastomosis was performed. Thereafter, a few to 10 episodes of bowel obstruction recurred each year, requiring hospitalization once or twice a year. To prevent bowel obstruction, he ate foods that had been processed with a blender.

Double-balloon endoscopy through the anus showed stenosis of the lower jejunum (Fig. 10.5.2a). A contrast-enhanced study with meglumine sodium amidotrizoate and the endoscope showed a filling defect around the endoscope tip (Fig. 10.5.2b), and a tattoo was placed near the stenotic site. Later, double-balloon endoscopy through the mouth revealed a tight bend of the lower jejunum, and the endoscope reached the tattoo placed caudal to the bend. The site was located in the center of the abdomen with no mobility and consistent

a 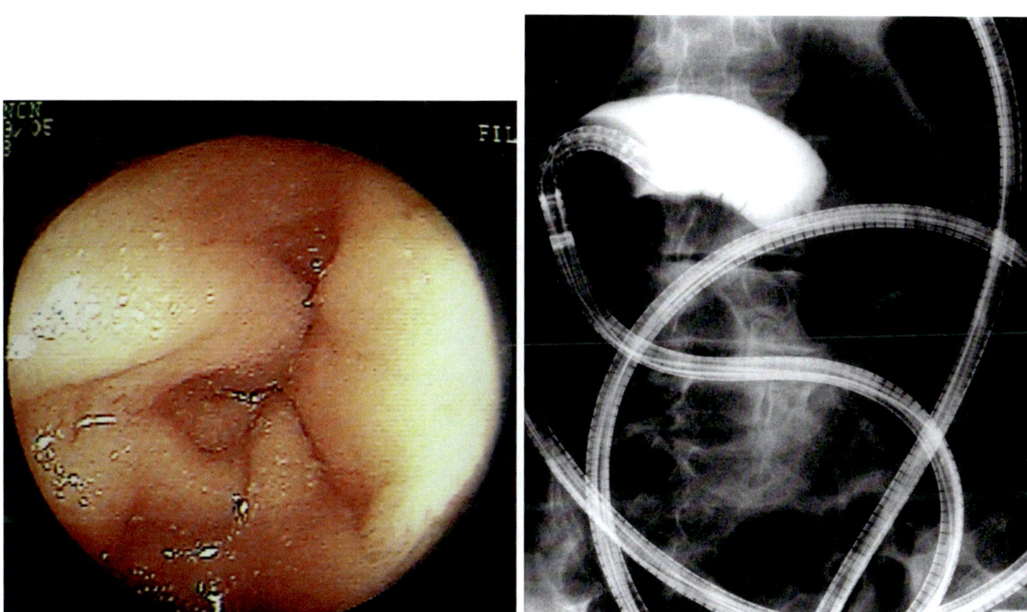 b

Fig. 10.5.2. Postoperative adhesive intestinal obstruction

a Stenosis by extrinsic compression revealed by double-balloon endoscopy through the anus

b No flow of contrast medium to the rostral side of the stenosis on a selective, contrast-enhanced radiograph (through the anus) with the surgical scar, leading to the conclusion that the site had resulted from adhesion to the abdominal wall (Fig. 10.5.2c). Computed tomography of the abdomen filled with gas revealed one adhesion to the abdominal wall in the subumbilical region (Fig. 10.5.2d), and laparoscopic division of adhesion was performed. As expected preoperatively, the adhesion was found rostral to the tattoo, which was divided (Fig. 10.5.2e). The tattoo was found near

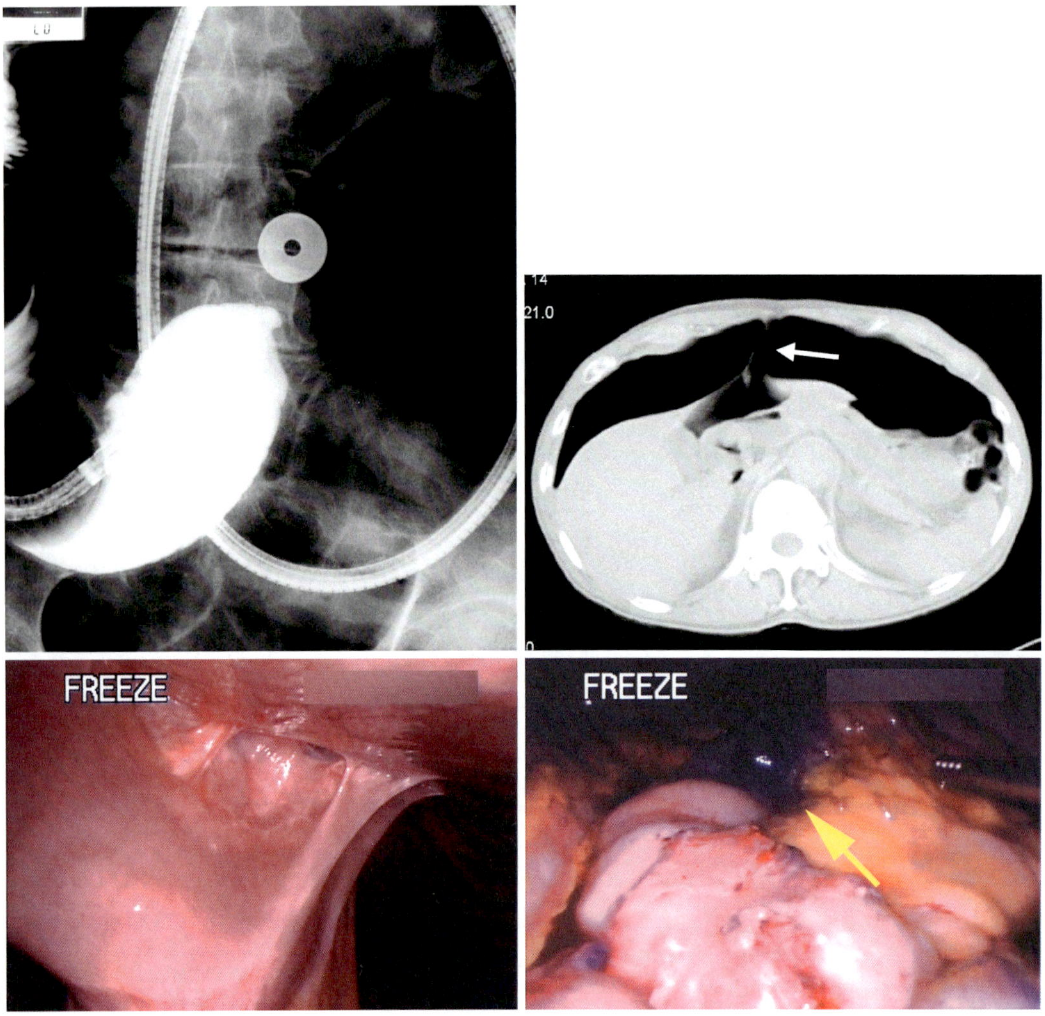

c d e f

Fig. 10.5.2. *continued.*

c Selective, contrast-enhanced radiograph (through the mouth), with the *round mark* indicating the umbilicus

d Computed tomography of the abdomen filled with gas revealed adhesion to the abdominal wall

e Adhesion found by laparoscopy

f Laparoscopic view after division of the adhesion. The arrow indicates the tatoo the divided site (Fig. 10.5.2f). He had a normal diet after division of the adhesion without recurrence of bowel obstruction symptoms.

Adhesive intestinal obstructions may be treated by laparotomy or laparoscopic surgery. Chopra et al. reported that laparoscopic surgery was useful and associated with less frequent complications, shorter operating time, and shorter length of hospital stay compared with laparotomy [2]. It is, however, difficult to locate precisely adhesions preoperatively. In some cases, laparoscopic surgery fails to identify the adhesion and stenosis and therefore has to be converted to laparotomy. As in this case, a tattoo placed at the stenotic site during double-balloon endoscopy serves as a useful mark for laparoscopic surgery. Preoperative double-balloon endoscopy is a therapeutic option in some patients undergoing elective division of adhesions.

References

1. Asakura H (1994) Blind loop syndrome. In: Domain specific syndrome series — gastrointestinal tract syndromes. Nippon Rinsho, Tokyo, pp 667–670
2. Chopra R, McVay C, Phillips E, et al (2003) Laparoscopic lysis of adhesions. Am Surg 69:966–968

10.6 Vascular Disease

Although relatively rare, vascular diseases in the intestine are clinically important because they may cause gastrointestinal bleeding. Common vascular diseases in the small intestine include angiodysplasia, arteriovenous malformation, hemangioma, and angiosarcoma (Table 10.6.1). Double-balloon endoscopy allows endoscopic observation of vascular diseases in the small intestine, which was previously difficult, and endoscopic interventions including hemostasis. Among vascular diseases in the small intestine, this subsection details angiodysplasia and hemangioma observed with the double-balloon endoscope.

10.6.1 Angiodysplasia

The term gastrointestinal angiodysplasia (see footnote) is conventionally used to describe angiectatic lesions localized in the gastrointestinal mucosa and submucosa. Angiodysplasia may occur in any portion of the stomach, small intestine, and large intestine. Angiodysplasia may cause gastrointestinal bleeding and should be taken into consideration as a differential diagnosis of gastrointestinal bleeding.

Table 10.6.1. Classification of vascular malformations and tumors and/or tumor-like lesions of the gastrointestinal tract

Vascular malformation
Angiodysplasia (vascular ectasia)
Arteriovenous malformation
Dieulafoy's vascular malformation
Vascular tumors and/or tumor-like lesions
Hemangioma
Capillary hemangioma
Cavernous hemangioma (single or diffuse)
Mixed capillary and cavernous hemangioma
Pyogenic granulomas (granulation tissue-type hemangioma)
Hemangiomatosis and specific vascular syndromes
Hemangiomatosis
Blue rubber bleb nevus syndrome
Hereditary hemorrhagic telangiectasia (Osler-Weber-Rendu disease)
Klippel-Trenaunay syndrome
Maffucci's syndrome
Diffuse intestinal (neonatal) hemangiomatosis
Angiosarcoma (malignant hemangioendothelioma)
Kaposi's sarcoma
Perivascular tumors
Benign tumors
Benign hemangiopericytoma
Glomus tumor
Malignant tumors
Malignant hemangiopericytoma

From Iwashita A, Oishi T, Yao T, et al. (2000) Pathological differential diagnosis of vascular diseases of gastrointestinal tract. Stomach Intestine (Tokyo) 35:774

Footnote: Angiodysplasia
According to the second edition of *Gastroenterological Endoscopy Terminology* (Tokyo: Igaku-Shion, 1997), the term "vascular malformation" or "angiodysplasia" was previously used to describe the lesion, which often causes lower gastrointestinal bleeding. However, the term "vascular ectasia" ("angiectasia" or "angiectasis") is more appropriate because the condition is attributable to vascular degeneration, an acquired cause.

● Case 1

A 31-year-old man with gastrointestinal bleeding underwent upper and lower endoscopy, which failed to identify the source of bleeding. Double-balloon endoscopy revealed angiodysplasia in the ileum (Fig. 10.6.1). About a dozen areas of angiodysplasia similar to that in the photograph were observed.

● Case 2

A 66-year-old woman with an unidentified source of gastrointestinal bleeding underwent double-balloon endoscopy, which revealed angiodysplasia in the jejunum (Fig. 10.6.2).

● Case 3

A 60-year-old woman underwent double-balloon endoscopy to investigate the cause of recurrent gastrointestinal bleeding. Multiple minute areas of angiodysplasia were found in the terminal ileum (Fig. 10.6.3).

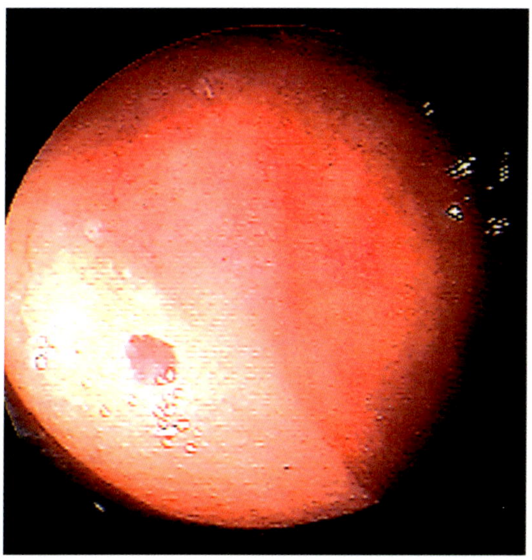

Fig. 10.6.1. Case 1. Angiodysplasia in the ileum

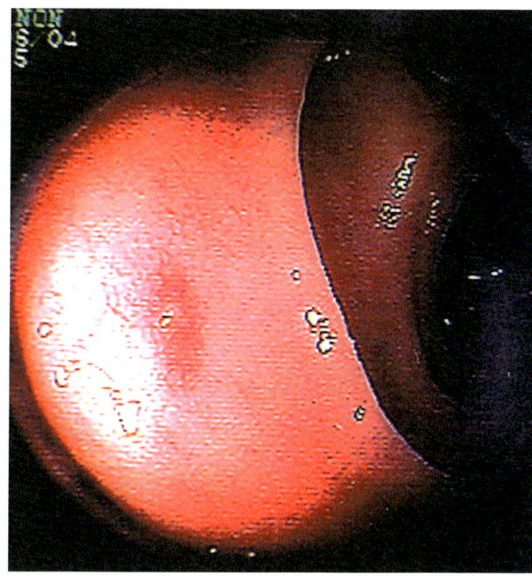

Fig. 10.6.2. Case 2. Angiodysplasia in the jejunum

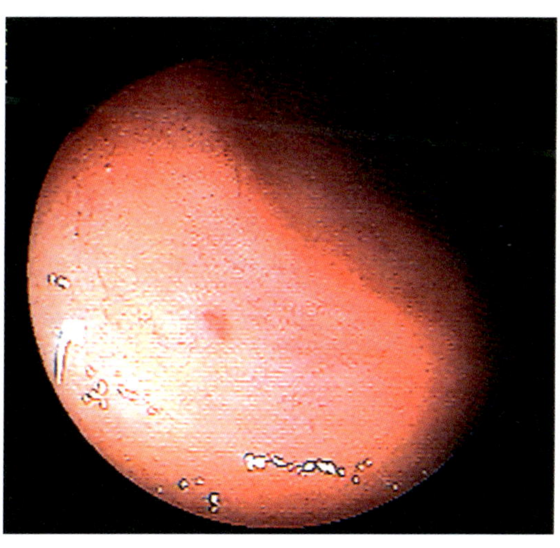

Fig. 10.6.3. Case 3. Minimal angiodysplasia in the terminal ileum

● Case 4

A 62-year-old woman was found to have angiodysplasia approximately 10 mm in size in the horizontal part of the duodenum (Fig. 10.6.4a). It was determined to be the cause of her gastrointestinal bleeding and was treated after observation. Physiological saline was injected under the mucosa of the lesion (Fig. 10.6.4b). Because the wall of the small intestine is thin, injection of physiological saline under the mucosa of the lesion is done to minimize the effect of coagulation on the muscle layer. The lesion immediately after cauterization with the tip of a snare is shown in Fig. 10.6.4c. Cauterization was performed with an ICC 200 (Erbe) in the soft coagulation mode at 60 W. The lesion was adequately cauterized. An endoscopic view of the lesion on day 8 after cauterization is presented in Fig. 10.6.4d. The lesion was adequately cauterized, and the patient recovered uneventfully.

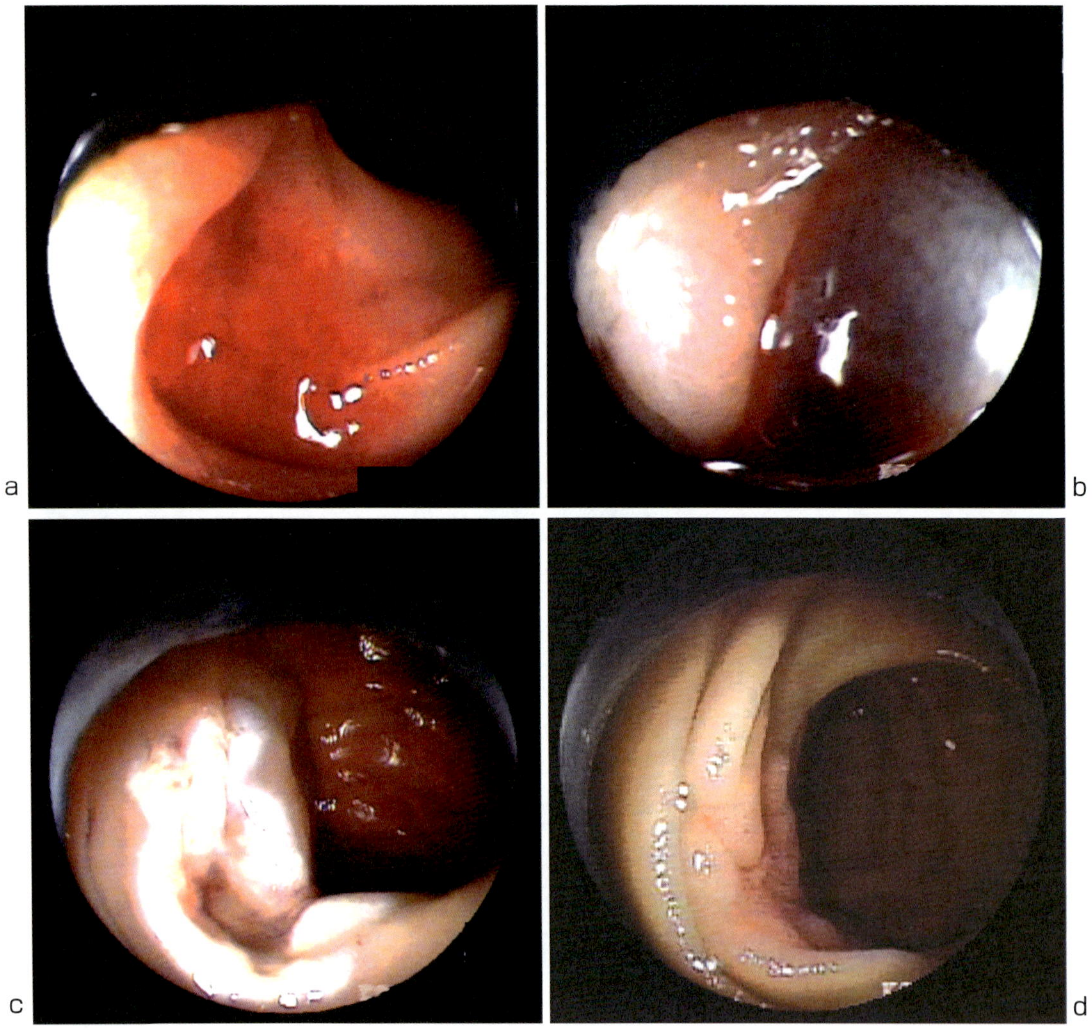

Fig. 10.6.4. Case 4

a Angiodysplasia approximately 10 mm in size in the horizontal part of the duodenum

b Injection of physiological saline

c Cauterization by electrocoagulation

d Postoperative day 8

● Case 5

A 62-year-old woman with chronic gastrointestinal bleeding of unknown cause underwent double-balloon endoscopy, which revealed active bleeding from an area of angiodysplasia localized slightly caudal to the ligament of Treitz (Fig. 10.6.5a). The bleeding point was more clearly shown by underwater examination (Fig. 10.6.5b). Underwater examination in combination with balloon inflation at the endoscope tip helps visualize those lesions and provides an effective means of observation. This technique allows detection of minimal bleeding that is difficult to identify by routine examination. Underwater observation is also useful after hemostasis. Figure 10.6.5c shows the result of underwater observation after treatment of the lesion. No active bleeding was found. Underwater observation is effective in investigating overt bleeding (Fig. 10.6.5b) as well as minimal bleeding from microlesions (Fig. 10.6.5d).

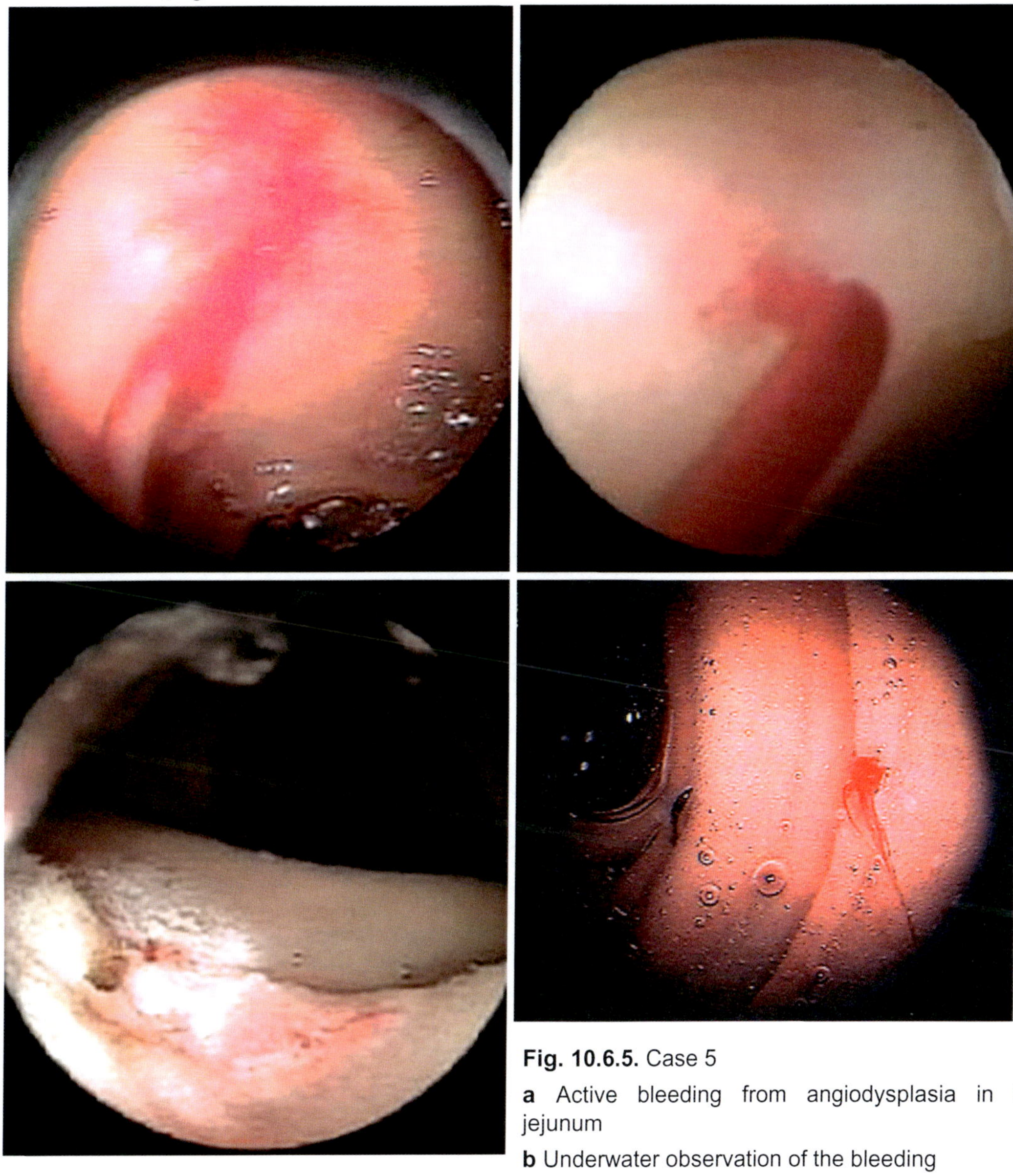

a b c d

Fig. 10.6.5. Case 5

a Active bleeding from angiodysplasia in the jejunum

b Underwater observation of the bleeding

c After electrocoagulation no active bleeding was found on underwater observation

d Underwater observation is effective for identifying bleeding from minimal lesions

10.6.2 Hemangioma

Hemangioma, a tumor consisting of proliferated blood vessels, occurs frequently in the skin but may develop in any part of the body, including the gastrointestinal tract. It has not been clearly determined whether hemangioma is a hamartoma, neoplasm, or deformity of existing blood vessels generated in response to chronic stimuli. Hemangioma may be found in the gastrointestinal tract of patients with congenital disorders, such as Osler-Weber-Rendu disease and Maffucci's syndrome.

● Case 6

A 41-year-old man with Maffucci's syndrome was diagnosed as having systemic multiple hemangioma, enchondroma, and chondrosarcoma in the head. Double-balloon endoscopy was performed because of recurrent gastrointestinal bleeding, and a hemangioma was found in the jejunum (Fig. 10.6.6). A small bowel series also showed multiple similarly protruding lesions.

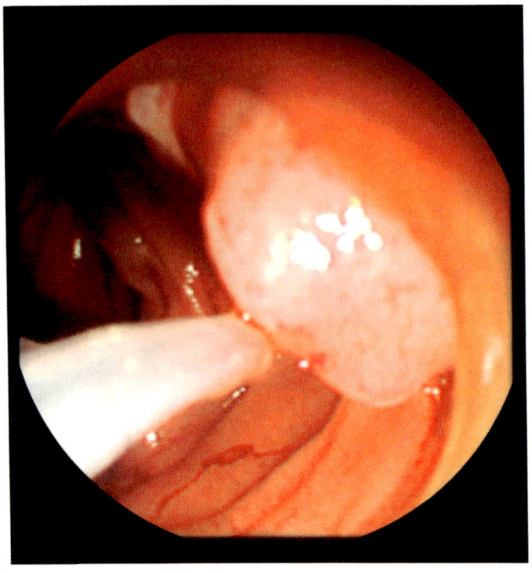

Fig. 10.6.6. Case 6. Hemangioma in the jejunum of a patient with Maffucci's syndrome

11 Endoscopic Treatment

11.1 Characteristics and Techniques of Endoscopic Treatment

11.1.1 Characteristics

Not only double-balloon endoscopy but other methods as well allow total enteroscopy. The most significant advantage of double-balloon endoscopy is its ability to make endoscopic treatment in the small intestine practical compared with other methods such as the sonde and ropeway methods and capsule endoscopy.

Like conventional upper endoscopes and colonoscopes, the double-balloon endoscope has a forceps channel through which therapeutic devices can be used. EN-450P5, an insertability-oriented, thin endoscope, has a forceps channel diameter of 2.2 mm and thus is limited regarding the use of therapeutic devices. The EN-450T5, a treatment type, has a 2.8-mm forceps channel and allows a variety of endoscopic interventions, including clipping.

Appropriate endoscopic interventions require an endoscope with excellent maneuverability and directionality. Even when an endoscope was successfully advanced into the distal small intestine by the conventional push method, it was sometimes difficult to perform interventions because of the instability of the endoscope tip. With double-balloon endoscopy, control of the endoscope is based on the fixed support established by the overtube balloon close to the lesion. This method thus allows excellent control and reliable manipulation of the endoscope even in the distal small intestine.

11.1.2 Techniques

It should be noted that the double-balloon endoscope—with its ability to be advanced to the affected region and subsequently removed with the overtube balloon secured near the affected region—substantially broadens the choice of therapeutic devices that can be used, which are conventionally limited by the forceps channel diameter and endoscope length. When used with the EN-450P5, therapeutic devices have to pass through a 2.2-mm forceps channel and the 230-cm endoscope. When the endoscope is removed, any device can be used so long as it can pass through the overtube (internal diameter 10 mm, total length 145 cm). Leaving the overtube in place facilitates reinsertion of the endoscope, thereby permitting endoscopic evaluation after the intervention. Changes in the type of endoscope with the overtube left in place may be useful for some interventions.

11.1.3 Therapeutic Devices Compatible with the Double-Balloon Endoscope

The EN-450P5 requires dedicated therapeutic devices because of the limitation of the forceps channel diameter (2.2 mm). The EN-450T5 has a 2.8-mm forceps channel and thus allows the use of any long therapeutic device for the large intestine (2.8 mm × 2.3 m or longer).

11.1.3.1 *Therapeutic Devices for EN-450P5*

1. Biopsy forceps: Fujinon-BF1824SF (Fig. 11.1.1). The biopsy forceps is used to obtain tissue specimens for histological examination.

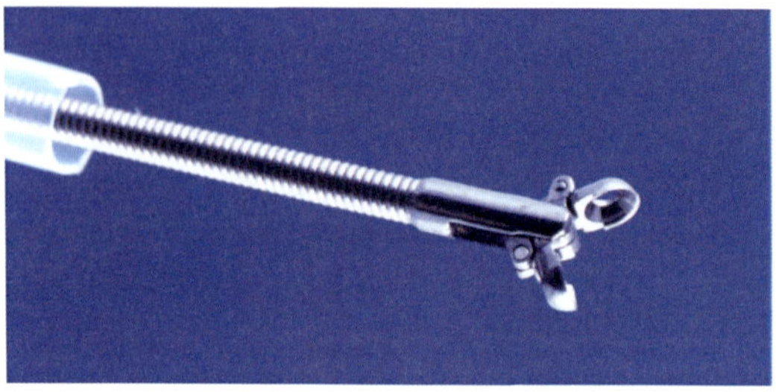

Fig. 11.1.1. Biopsy forceps: Fujinon-BF1824SF

2. Grasping forceps (three-nail type): Fujinon-GF1824T (Fig. 11.1.2). The grasping forceps is used to retrieve polyps and to hold foreign bodies.

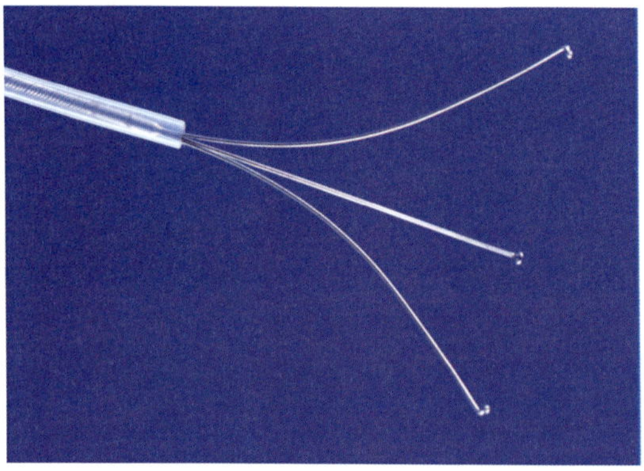

Fig. 11.1.2. Grasping forceps (three-nail type): Fujinon-GF1824T

3. High-frequency snare: Fujinon-DS1824H (Fig. 11.1.3). This is a high-frequency snare used for polypectomy and endoscopic mucosa resection (EMR).

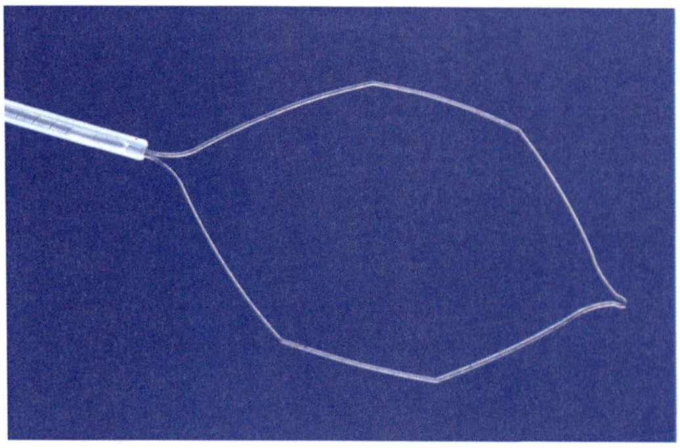

Fig. 11.1.3. High-frequency snare: Fujinon-DS1824H

4. Needle: Fujinon-IN1823MM34N6 (Fig. 11.1.4) The needle is used for submucosal injection during EMR, injection to stop bleeding, and tattooing.

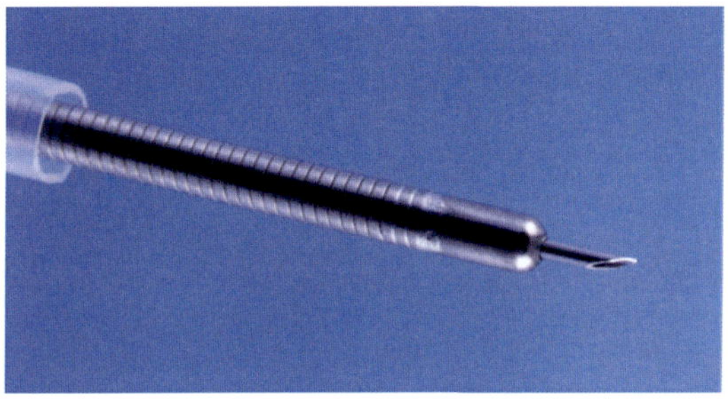

Fig. 11.1.4. Needle: Fujinon-IN1823MM34N6

5. Coagulation probe: Fujinon-DC1824R (Fig. 11.1.5). This is a monopolar probe for high-frequency electrocoagulation to stop bleeding. It allows effective hemostasis in soft coagulation mode.

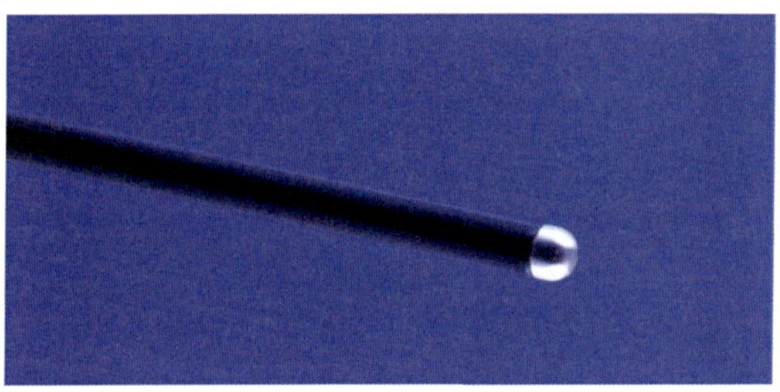

Fig. 11.1.5. Coagulation probe: Fujinon -DC1824R

6. Hot biopsy: Fujinon-DP1824HB (Fig. 11.1.6). This is a hot biopsy forceps for small polyps. Because of its small cups, it is also used safely as a hemostatic forceps.

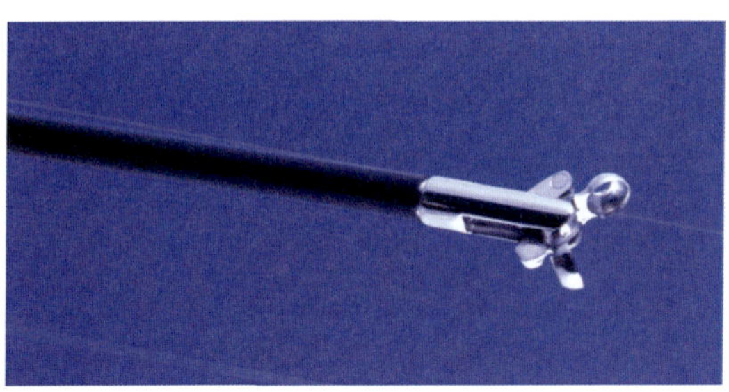

Fig. 11.1.6. Hot biopsy: Fujinon-DP1824HB

11.1.3.2 Representative Useful Therapeutic Devices for Use with EN-450T5

1. Endoscopic clip. Resolution Clip 2261 (Boston Scientific) (Fig. 11.1.7) and disposable Quick Clip HX-200U-135 (Olympus) (Fig. 11.1.8) are available.

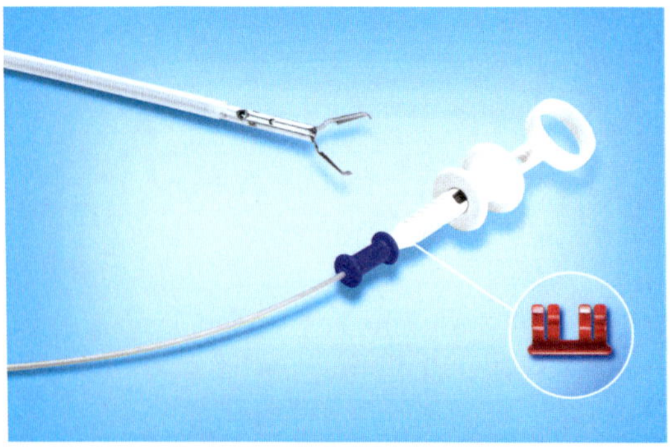

Fig. 11.1.7. Resolution Clip 2261 (Boston Scientific)

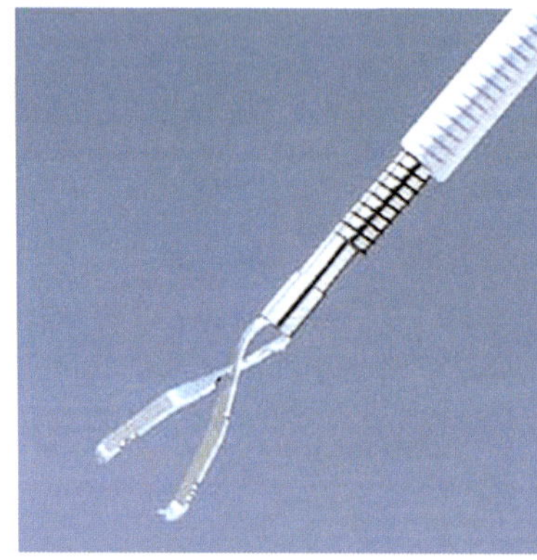

Fig. 11.1.8. Quick Clip HX-200U-135 (Olympus)

2. Argon plasma coagulation device. Argon plasma coagulation (APC) probes 20132-179 and 20132-166 (Erbe) (Fig. 11.1.9) are available, which are useful for coagulation of angiodysplasia.

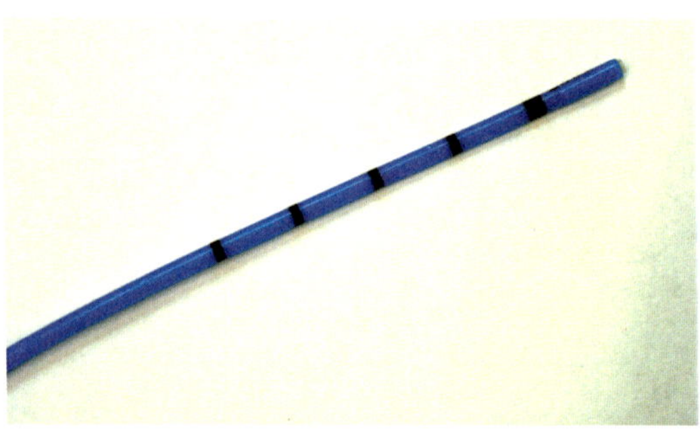

Fig. 11.1.9. Argon plasma coagulation (APC) probe 20132-179, 20132-166 (Erbe)

3. Endoscope balloon dilator. Balloon dilator CRE WG (colonic) is available (Boston Scientific) (Fig. 11.1.10).

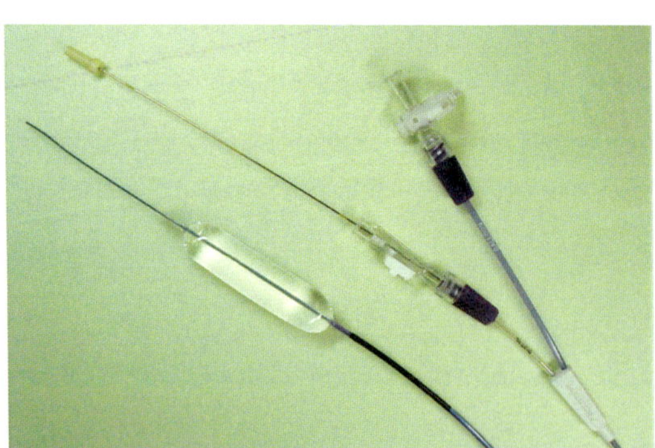

Fig. 11.1.10. CRE WG (colonic) (Boston Scientific)

11.2 Hemostasis

11.2.1 Small-Intestinal Bleeding

Bleeding lesions may be found in the small intestine as well as other portions of the gastrointestinal tract, some of which require urgent treatment in clinical settings. Even if a patient's condition necessitates resecting the stomach or large intestine, the patient can be rehabilitated to lead a normal social life, although some gastrointestinal symptoms may occur after surgery. However, the small intestine plays a life-sustaining role of digestion and absorption. If resection of the small intestine is required in a patient with small-intestinal bleeding, the patient will suffer from short bowel syndrome for the rest of his or her life after surgery unless the resection is kept to a minimum to maintain the remaining intestinal function.

With small-intestinal bleeding, however, identifying the bleeding site is generally difficult. In the case of massive bleeding, urgent laparotomy may be performed to resect a large amount of the small intestine, including the region with blood retention; or the bleeding site can be identified by angiography and its affected region, revealed by dye injection, resected. Both methods necessitate resection of a large amount of the intestine. With gastrointestinal bleeding, a bleeding point is usually found on the luminal side of the gastrointestinal tract. The full use of the double-balloon endoscope allows physicians to pinpoint the bleeding site in the intestinal lumen rather than approximate the site. Use of the double-balloon endoscope allows precise localization of bleeding sites in the small intestine and successful endoscopic hemostasis, thereby obviating surgery. In cases where endoscopic hemostasis is difficult, a tattoo placed on the luminal side allows identification of the bleeding site in the small intestine from the serosal side, thereby minimizing the extent of resection if intestinal resection is needed later.

11.2.2 Endoscopic Treatment of Small-Intestinal Bleeding

Various methods of endoscopic hemostasis have been developed for successful treatment of a variety of bleeding lesions in the gastrointestinal tract, including a peptic ulcer in the stomach and duodenum and angiodysplasia and diverticular hemorrhage in the large intestine. These successful endoscopic treatments obviate surgery in many patients, and endoscopic hemostasis is one of the great achievements of therapeutic endoscopy. A variety of hemostatic techniques, including injection of ethanol or hypertonic saline, cauterization with an argon plasma coagulator (APC) or a heat probe, and hemostasis with a clip have been developed and put to practical use. They have led to the establishment of therapeutics involving the selection, indications, and techniques of treatments based on the pathological condition of the bleeding lesions. Although the principle of insertion differs between the double-balloon endoscope and conventional endoscopes, all hemostatic techniques used for conventional upper and lower endoscopy are applicable to treatment using the double-balloon endoscope. However, endoscopic hemostasis with the double-balloon endoscope requires consideration of three factors.

The first factor is the anatomical characteristics of the small intestine, and the second is the pathophysiology of the bleeding lesion(s) in the small intestine. The third factor is the limitation intrinsic to the endoscopic system, such as the EN-450P5 with a working length of 200 cm and a forceps channel diameter of 2.2 mm. This problem has been resolved by the treatment-type endoscope EN-450T5 with a 2.8-mm forceps channel.

Anatomically, the intestinal wall is thin. Particularly when thermocoagulation is chosen for hemostasis, then, the risk of perforation increases as coagulation depth increases. Because of limitations on the therapeutic devices that can be used with the EN-450P5, we used the tip of a snare to perform coagulation and hemostasis for the treatment of many bleeding lesions. In cases of bleeding from the center of tumors such as the gastrointestinal stromal tumor (GIST), adequate cauterization can be achieved with less consideration of coagulation depth. In cases of bleeding from angiodysplasia, saline is injected submucosally under lesions to provide substantial mucosal elevation, and then hemostasis is performed with due attention given to the coagulation depth.

The second consideration is the pathophysiology of bleeding lesions in the small intestine. The usefulness of identifying an exposed vessel and the technique for accurate hemostasis of the exposed vessel have been demonstrated for peptic ulcers in the stomach and the duodenal bulb. Various conditions, such as Crohn's disease, Behçet's disease, and nonsteroidal antiinflammatory drug (NSAID) use, may induce ulceration in the small intestine. We rarely have identified and treated exposed vessels in patients with intestinal ulcers associated with these pathological conditions. However, intestinal Behçet's disease is often associated with deep ulcers, which can result in massive bleeding that necessitates emergency surgery. Similarly, Crohn's disease may lead to massive bleeding. Thus, treatment of ulcerative lesions requires the establishment of diagnostics to evaluate the depth and appearance of ulcers and to assess the bleeding risk, as well as therapeutic techniques for visible vessels if identified. Angiodysplasia tends to occur at multiple sites, and active bleeding found on examination is regarded as the source of bleeding. Otherwise, it cannot be determined whether the identified lesion is responsible for the bleeding. In those cases, lesions with or without active bleeding are cauterized when possible. Thus, it is necessary to establish safe, reliable therapeutic techniques taking into consideration the thinness of the small-intestinal wall, as described above. An APC probe is compatible with EN-450T5, and cauterization by APC can go mainstream as in the stomach and the large intestine. Bleeding lesions in the small intestine often occur at multiple sites, and well-planned enteroscopy is often needed to examine the entire small intestine.

The third consideration comprises the limitations intrinsic to the system, such as the EN-450P5 with a working length of 200 cm and a forceps channel diameter of 2.2 mm. We previously used the tip of a snare as a thermocoagulation device, but the development of APC probes has increased our options on therapeutic devices. The treatment-type endoscope EN-450T5 with a 2.8-mm forceps channel is now commercially available and allows the use of clips and hemostatic forceps. We take into consideration the risk of tissue injury and do not use ethanol or hypertonic saline in principle.

Advice

Tips for Tattooing with an Endoscope

Successful submucosal injection is difficult because an injection needle easily penetrates the muscle layer of the thin small-intestinal wall. If the India ink used for tattooing leaks into the lumen, visibility worsens. These problems may be solved by the following strategies. First, the injection needle is filled with physiological saline instead of India ink. After physiological saline is injected to elevate the mucosa and the needle tip is securely placed in the submucosal layer, the syringe is replaced with another syringe filled with India ink, and the ink is then injected with the same needle tip. The injection needle is removed while slight negative pressure is applied to prevent leakage of India ink.

● Case 1
Saline injection and subsequent coagulation and hemostasis for the treatment of active bleeding from angiodysplasia in the small intestine (Figs. 11.2.1, 11.2.2).

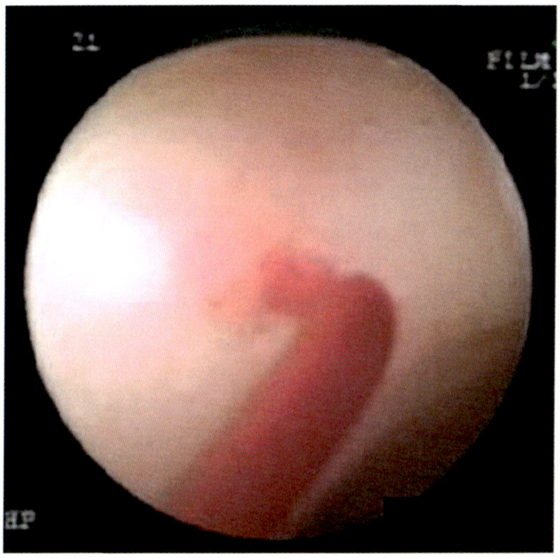
Fig. 11.2.1. Active bleeding from angiodysplasia

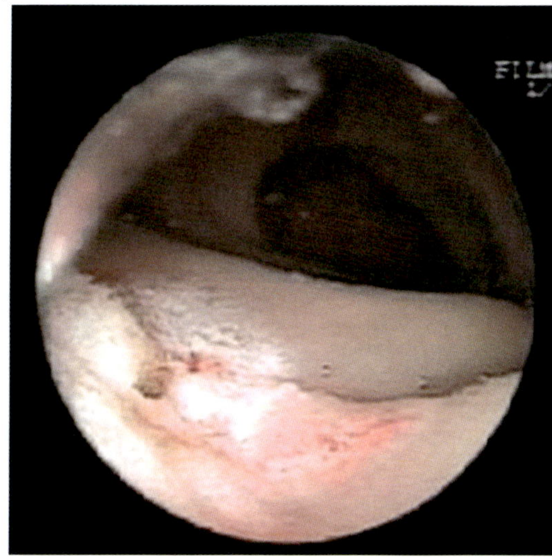
Fig. 11.2.2. Hemostasis for angiodysplasia

● Case 2
Coagulation and hemostasis for the treatment of bleeding from a small-intestinal tumor (Figs. 11.2.3, 11.2.4).

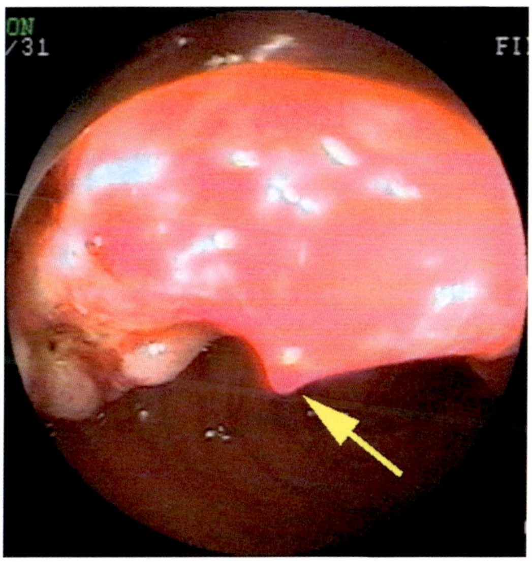
Fig. 11.2.3. Active bleeding from a small-intestinal tumor

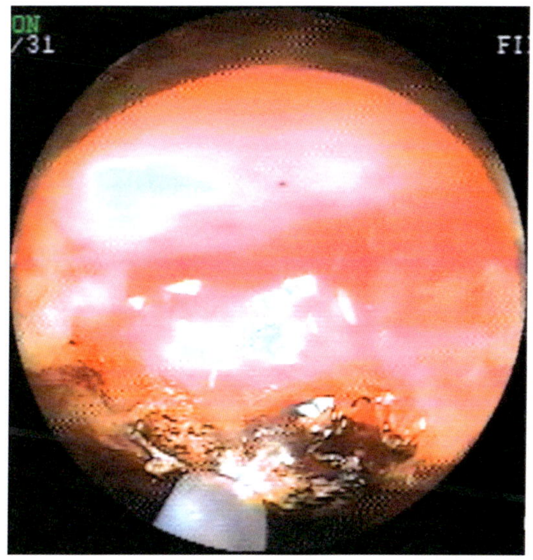
Fig. 11.2.4. Hemostasis for the treatment of bleeding from a small-intestinal tumor

11.3 Polypectomy and Endoscopic Mucosal Resection

The conventional push enteroscopy does not allow an endoscope to advance more than 1 m distal to the ligament of Treitz, and polypectomy cannot be performed in the small intestine beyond this limit. Even in a small intestine accessible to the endoscope, it is often difficult to perform a safe, reliable polypectomy of intestinal polyps because of a stretched intestine and poor maneuverability of the endoscope. Double-balloon endoscopy provides good maneuverability of the endoscope even in the distal small intestine because intestinal stretching is prevented and the endoscope is supported by the tip of the overtube during insertion. These advantages enable polypectomy and other interventions that require close observation and fine manipulation even in the small intestine similar to that in upper endoscopy and colonoscopy.

11.3.1 Indications

Hyperplastic polyps, neoplastic polyps (adenoma, carcinoma), hamartomatous polyps, and inflammatory polyps may occur in the small intestine. Hyperplastic and inflammatory polyps are indications for polypectomy if they pose a risk of bleeding or intussusception. In contrast to adenomas of the large intestine, the adenoma-carcinoma sequence has not been established in the small intestine, and consensus has not been reached about the indications for polypectomy. Some favor polypectomy considering the difficulty of regular follow-up with upper and lower endoscopy. Investigation of melena or hematochezia with an unidentified source of bleeding may reveal a bleeding polyp, which is the best indication for a polypectomy (case 1).

11.3.2 Technique

First, the polyp of interest should be fully observed. After mucus is cleared, the shape, color, tension, and condition around the mucosa are observed in a way similar to colonoscopic observation. Because the Fujinon double-balloon electronic endoscope has a forceps channel at the 7 o'clock position, the lesion should be located at the 7 o'clock position on the monitor. When the overtube is securely placed, it is easy to rotate the double-balloon endoscope unless the endoscope forms an intricate loop such as a sigmoid shape. The patient's posture may be adjusted so the endoscope is advanced to an appropriate place for easy treatment. When a polyp is localized in a bend, slight withdrawal of the endoscope together with the overtube fixed to the intestinal wall may straighten the distal small intestine and improve the view.

When resection is indicated and deemed safe, prepare for polypectomy. In the small intestine, a histologically normal mucosa is as thin as approximately 200–400 μm (excluding the thickness of the villi), and the muscularis mucosae is 40 μm in thickness (the mucosa is 1 mm and the muscularis mucosae 100 μm in the stomach; the mucosa is 600 μm and the muscularis mucosae 50 μm in the large intestine). Because the intestinal wall is thin, direct snaring and cautery resection could coagulate the muscularis propria and cause perforation. Even if perforation does not occur immediately, necrosis of the muscularis propria caused by excess current flow may result in perforation 1–2 days after coagulation (delayed perforation). Thus, we perform submucosal saline injection and then snaring and EMR to resect lesions, including subpedunculated polyps, to avoid spreading excess heat to the muscularis propria and accidentally snaring the muscularis propria.

11.3.3 Complications

Bleeding and perforation may occur after polypectomy same as in the large intestine. We had a case of mild bleeding after polypectomy that stopped spontaneously within 2 days. If bleeding occurs and the intestinal tract is filled with a large amount of blood, it is difficult to reinsert the double-balloon endoscopy. If the endoscope is successfully reinserted to identify the bleeding site, injection of epinephrine-containing saline, high-frequency coagulation such as APC, and clipping can be performed for hemostasis. Minor bleeding (with a minimal decrease in the hemoglobin level) may be stopped with conservative treatment. For perforation in the stomach, endoscopic closure of the lesion with clips and conservative treatment are commonly performed [1]. In the large intestine, closure with clips and conservative treatment may be sufficient for pinhole-sized perforations associated with endoscopic submucosal dissection. Because of the presence of many bacteria in the large intestine, however, laparoscopic or laparotomic intraperitoneal irrigation and drainage should be considered in patients with leakage of intestinal fluids and resultant peritoneal irritation symptoms and fever [2]. We have not encountered small-intestinal perforations after a polypectomy; if such a perforation occurs, it should be treated with endoscopic clipping or laparoscopic or laparotomic wound closure and irrigation drainage, similar to that for large-intestinal perforation.

11.3.4 Methods for Collecting Resected Lesions

11.3.4.1 *Suction*

With colonoscopy, a small polyp ($\leq$ 5 mm) is often collected by direct suctioning through the forceps channel. The enteroscope, with a 2.2-mm forceps channel, allows suction of a small polyp ($\leq$ 3 mm) into a trap. The EN-450T5, with a 2.8-mm forceps channel, permits collection of larger polyps through the forceps channel. A large polyp 5 mm or more can be securely attached to the endoscope tip by suction and then collected by withdrawing the endoscope with the overtube left in position. When an endoscope with a hood attached is withdrawn, the hood at the endoscope tip falls off. Consequently, the hood should be collected with a basket forceps (described later). The endoscope should be inserted without a hood when a polyp $\geq$ 5 mm is to be excised (see Chapter 7).

11.3.4.2 *Basket Forceps and Retrieval Net*

The basket forceps used with a cholangioscope (FG-33W, Olympus) has a working length of 2500 mm and an outer diameter of 1.7 mm; it is fully compatible with the EN-450P5/20 with a forceps channel diameter of 2.2 mm. Because of its small basket, however, the forceps cannot securely hold an object larger than 10 mm even when the basket is opened to the maximum. The treatment-type EN-450T5 endoscope with a forceps channel diameter of 2.8 mm allows the use of a basket forceps (FU-16U-1) for colonoscopes and retrieval of an object up to approximately 20 mm. The EN-450T5 also allows use of a disposable retrieval net (product no. 711182) with which an object 20 mm in size can be retrieved.

11.3.5 Case Presentation

● Case 1

A 58-year-old woman with chronic, progressive anemia was referred to our hospital by a local physician. Capsule endoscopy revealed a bleeding polyp-like lesion around the jejunoileal junction. Double-balloon endoscopy performed through the mouth showed an erythematous subpedunculated polyp 5 mm in diameter near the upper ileum (Fig. 11.3.1a). After saline injection, EMR was performed. The polyp was resected without considerable bleeding or other complications, and the site was marked with India ink (Fig. 11.3.1b) [3].

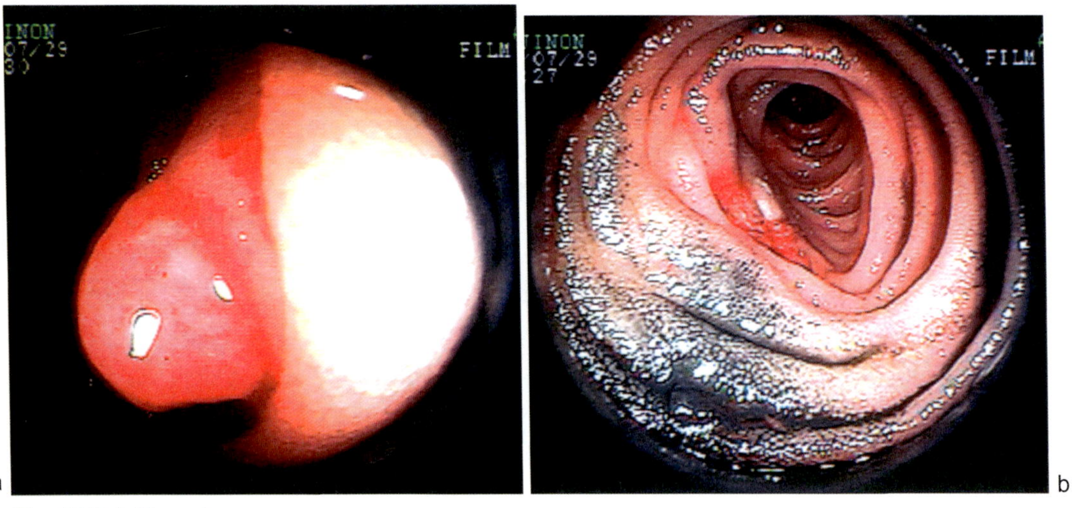

a b

Fig. 11.3.1. Case 1

a Polyp 5 mm in diameter

b After resection, a tattoo was placed rostral to the lesion

● Case 2

A 69-year-old man with previous Roux-en-Y reconstruction for gastric cancer was referred for investigation of eosinophilia and chronic diarrhea. The double-balloon endoscope advanced through the Roux-en-Y anastomosis to the blind end of the afferent loop. In addition to the papilla of Vater, a protruding lesion was found at the blind end of the afferent loop (Fig. 11.3.2a,b). Biopsy findings suggested adenocarcinoma. Thus, double-balloon endoscopy was repeated for EMR. A 70-cm short overtube was advanced to the lesion of interest and secured in place (Fig. 11.3.2d-1,2d-2). The endoscope was removed with the overtube left in place, and a thin upper endoscope with a larger forceps channel was inserted (Fig. 11.3.2d-3,2d-4). After saline injection, EMR was performed (Fig. 11.3.2c). The pathology examination led to a diagnosis of well-differentiated adenocarcinoma (IIa, sm1) with clear margins [4]. The patient was treated with the EN-450P5 before development of the EN-450T5; the use of the EN-450T5 obviates switching endoscopes.

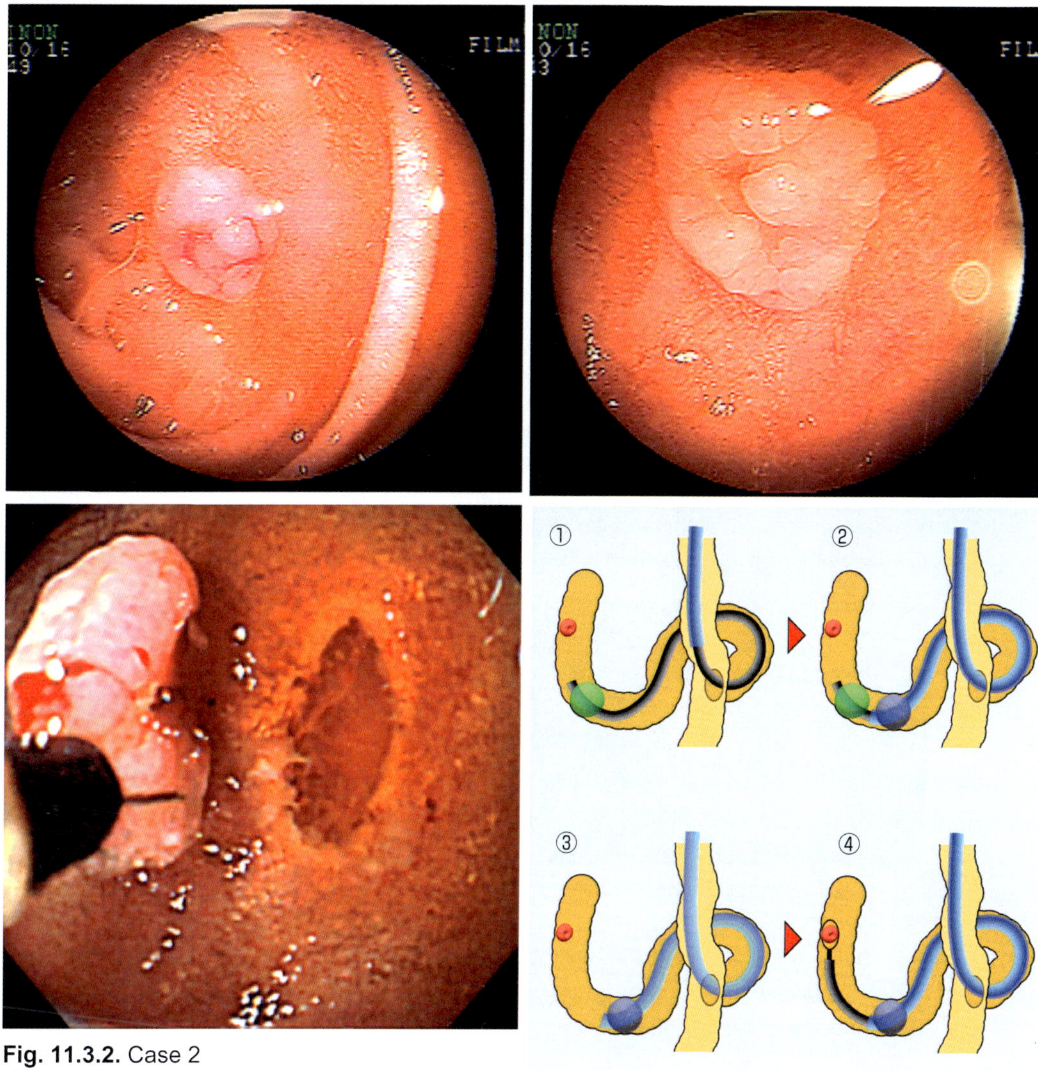

Fig. 11.3.2. Case 2

a Protruding lesion in the blind end of the afferent loop

b Close-up of the lesion in **a**

c Endoscopic mucosal resection of the entire lesion

d Technical procedure

References

1. Ono H (2002) Treatment of perforation occurring during EMR for gastroduodenal disease. Endosc Dig 2:187–192
2. Yamamoto H (2002) Complications of endoscopic treatment—perforations during therapeutic colonoscopy. Early Colorectal Cancer 6:129–134
3. Kita H, Yamamoto H, Nakamura T, et al (2005) Bleeding polyp in the mid small intestine identified by capsule endoscopy and treated by double-balloon endoscopy. Gastrointest Endosc 61:628–629
4. Kuno A, Yamamoto H, Kita H, et al (2004) Application of double-balloon enteroscopy through Roux-en-Y anastomosis for the endoscopic mucosal resection of an early carcinoma in the duodenal afferent limb. Gastrointest Endosc 60:1032–1034

11.4 Balloon Dilatation and Stenting

The treatment-type double-balloon endoscope (EN-450T5) has the same working length (200 cm) as the observation type (EN-450P5/20) but a larger forceps channel of 2.8 mm; it therefore allows interventions with an endoscopic balloon dilator, as performed with the conventional endoscope (Fig. 11.4.1). However, it can be used not only for balloon dilatation but also for hemostasis by clipping or APC. In contrast, the observation-type double-balloon endoscope (EN-450P5/20) has a narrow forceps channel of 2.2 mm, and a balloon dilator for the conventional endoscope therefore cannot be inserted through the forceps channel. After advancing the endoscope to the affected region, however, one can perform interventions under fluoroscopic guidance by withdrawing the endoscope and leaving the balloon-attached overtube (internal diameter 10 mm, total length 145 cm) (hereafter referred to as the overtube) in the intestine, thereby establishing a short, straightened route to the affected region. In addition, the "endoscope removal method" unique to double-balloon endoscopy may even be applied to place a stent in the small intestine. This subsection details the endoscopic treatment of stenosis of the small intestine.

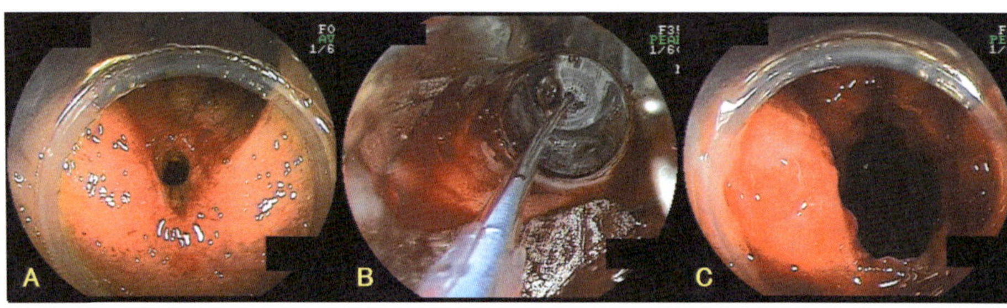

Fig. 11.4.1. Balloon dilatation with the treatment-type double-balloon endoscope (EN-450T5)

A Stenosis of the small intestine associated with Crohn's disease

B Balloon dilatation while monitoring the stenotic site through the balloon

C Stenotic site after dilatation

11.4.1 Balloon Dilatation of the Stenotic Site by the Endoscope Removal Method: Procedure

1. Instead of a fixing rubber, nylon surgical sutures (3-0 or 4-0 in size) or nylon fishing line (approximately 0.145 mm in diameter, equivalent to no. 0.8) is used to secure the endoscope balloon (Fig. 11.4.2). In this situation, a hood is not attached to the endoscope. When the hood is absolutely necessary for insertion of the endoscope, the hood is mounted (not secured with surgical tape). It should be noted that the hood must be left in the intestine when the endoscope is removed. It is retrieved endoscopically at the end of the intervention or is excreted in the feces (see section 11.4.3 for the method of collecting the hood) (Fig. 11.4.2).

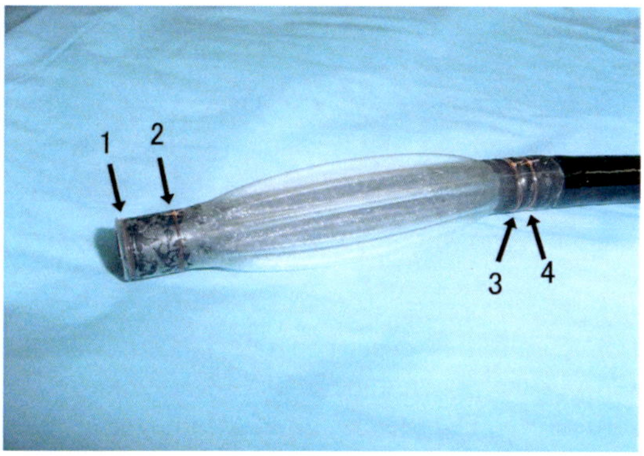

Fig. 11.4.2. Securing the endoscope balloon with sutures

Four sites should be secured. The second ligature from the tip must be placed distal to the opening of the air route on the lateral side of the tip. Without the second ligature, a deflated endoscope balloon may limit the field of view during examination

2. The double-balloon endoscope is used to locate the stenotic site in the small intestine and to determine the length and number of the stenotic sites with a water-soluble contrast agent (Figs. 11.4.3, 11.4.4).

Figs. 11.4.3 to 11.4.8 are from the same patient.

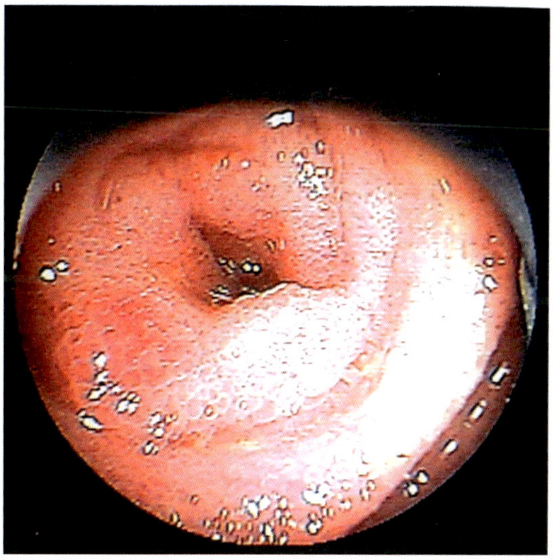

Fig. 11.4.3. Delayed ileal stenosis after blunt abdominal trauma in a 42-year-old man

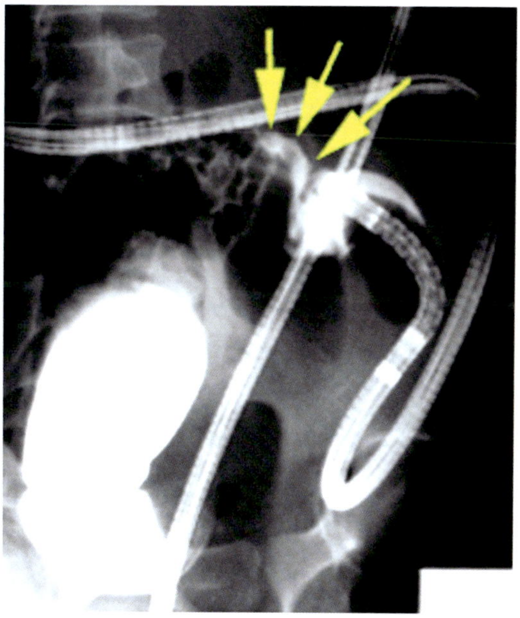

Fig. 11.4.4. Selective, contrast-enhanced radiograph

Selective, contrast-enhanced radiograph showing a stenosis (*arrows*) approximately 1 cm in length together with distension of the proximal portion of the intestine (the endoscope was inserted through the anus)

3. A guidewire (0.35 mm diameter, 450 cm length) (Jagwire) is inserted through the forceps channel of the endoscope and placed beyond the stenotic site. The endoscope is then removed, leaving the guidewire and the overtube in the small intestine (Fig. 11.4.5). A hood, if attached, drops off at this point.

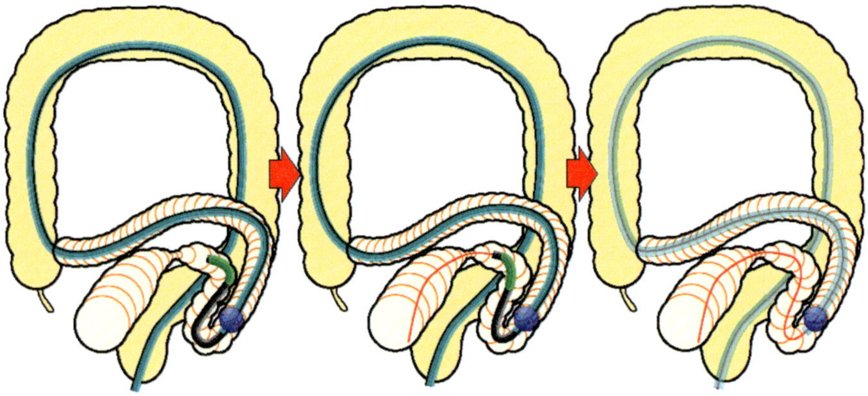

Fig. 11.4.5. A guidewire is placed beyond the stenotic site, and the endoscope alone is removed

4. A 150-cm plastic tube (whose preparation is described later) is inserted along the guidewire and the overtube. The tip of the plastic tube is placed just short of the tip of the overtube under fluoroscopic guidance. The plastic tube facilitates smooth insertion of a balloon dilator. The dilatation balloon with an expended diameter of 8–15 mm is inserted along the guidewire, plastic tube, and overtube to the affected region to dilate the stenotic site. An appropriate balloon is chosen based on the length of the stenotic site (Fig. 11.4.6; see also Fig.11.4.7).

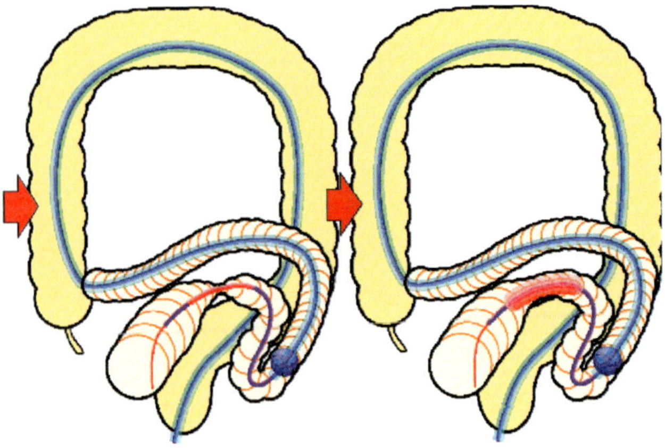

Fig. 11.4.6. A balloon dilator is used to dilate the stenotic site

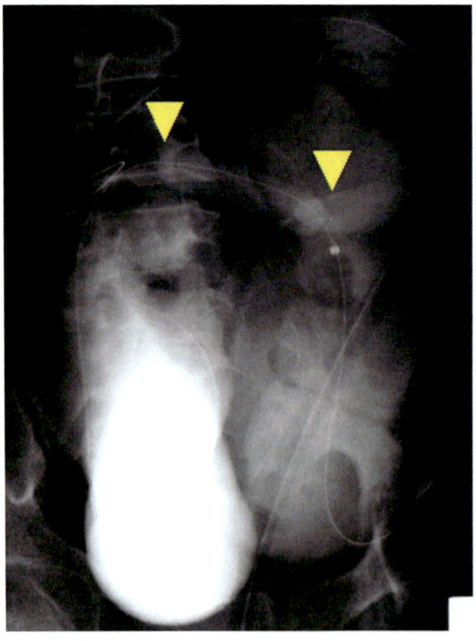

Fig. 11.4.7. Selective, contrast-enhanced radiograph during balloon inflation

The *arrowheads* indicate the two ends of the balloon

5. The balloon is then deflated. The degree of dilatation is evaluated, and the balloon is inflated again as appropriate. The balloon dilator may be replaced with a different size of dilatation balloon with the plastic tube in place. If a contrast agent is injected into the proximal opening of the overtube, an additional contrast-enhanced study can be performed during the intervention (Fig. 11.4.8). After completing the dilatation, the dilatation balloon, guidewire, and plastic tube are removed through the overtube. Reinserting the endoscope into the overtube, which is placed to shorten and straighten the intestine, allows easy endoscopic evaluation of the efficacy of the dilatation immediately after intervention.

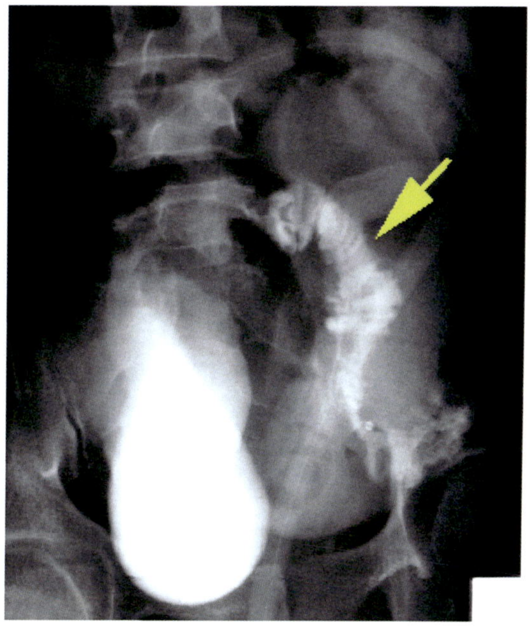

Fig. 11.4.8. Selective, contrast-enhanced radiograph after balloon dilatation

Intestinal contents retained in the proximal portion passed through (*arrow*) immediately after dilatation

11.4.2 Application to Stenting for Stenosis

By applying the aforementioned balloon dilatation technique, we successfully placed a metal stent for circumferential stenosis associated with inoperable jejunal malignancy. A 65-year-old woman with primary jejunal carcinoma and multiple hepatic metastases was referred to our hospital for treatment of bowel obstruction. On presentation, the patient had not eaten for a long time. Bypass surgery was initially considered to improve her quality of life, but she refused to undergo laparotomy and insisted on endoscopic treatment. Thus, we located the stenotic site in the jejunum by double-balloon endoscopy and applied the aforementioned balloon dilatation technique to place an esophageal stent (Ultraflex, Boston Scientific) at the stenotic site. She resumed oral food intake immediately after stenting, and bowel obstruction did not recur until she died about 1.5 months later (Figs. 11.4.9–11.4.12).

Advice

Points to Consider Regarding Balloon Dilatation

For smooth insertion of a therapeutic device, the intestinal route to the affected region is preferably well shortened. Considerable caution should be observed to avoid intestinal perforation, and balloon dilatation should be performed in a stepwise fashion under fluoroscopic guidance.

Advice

Points to Consider in the Presence of Multiple Stenotic Sites

If the initial contrast-enhanced study shows multiple stenotic sites in a short segment, a guidewire is preferably advanced through as many stenotic sites as possible at a time. This allows consecutive dilatation of multiple stenotic sites with a dilatation balloon, thereby reducing the intervention time.

Advice

Tips for Injection with the Double-Balloon Endoscope

The double-balloon endoscope has a thin forceps channel and a working length of 200 cm, which is longer than the conventional endoscope, thereby requiring a thin, long injection needle. Such a needle is generally floppy, and it is sometimes difficult to advance it through the forceps channel to the tip. To solve this problem, it is recommended that a trace amount of olive oil be injected into the forceps channel before inserting an injection needle. A stylet used with an injection needle should be removed after the injection needle is found to come out of the endoscope tip, followed by filling in the injection needle.

Figs. 11.4.9 to 11.4.12 are from the same patient.

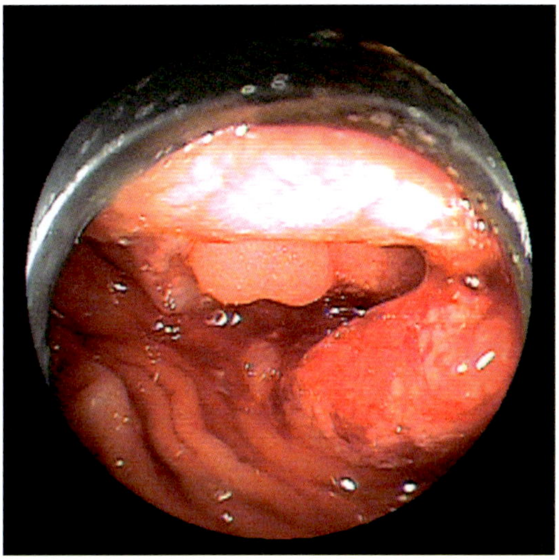

Fig. 11.4.9. Circumferential stenosis associated with jejunal carcinoma

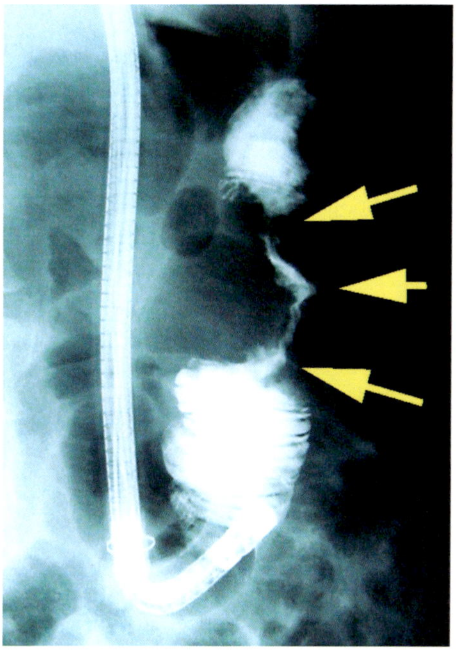

Fig. 11.4.10. Selective, contrast-enhanced radiograph

Selective, contrast-enhanced radiograph showing a stenotic site (*arrows*)

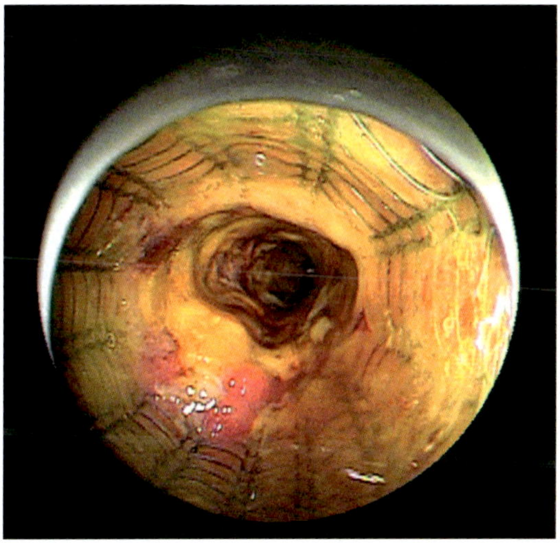

Fig. 11.4.11. Double-balloon endoscopy performed 5 days later

Stent patency was demonstrated

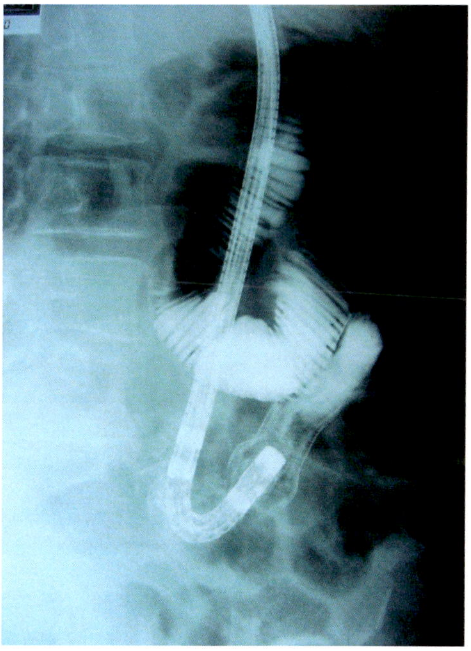

Fig. 11.4.12. Selective, contrast-enhanced radiograph obtained at the same time as Fig. 11.4.11

Selective, contrast-enhanced radiograph obtained at the same time as Fig. 11.4.11 demonstrated substantial flow of a contrast agent to the anal side and stent patency

11.4.3 Retrieval of Dropped Hood

Whereas a hood left caudal to the stenotic site is spontaneously excreted in the feces, a hood left proximal to the site may be retained in the gastrointestinal tract as a foreign body. Spontaneous excretion is unlikely, particularly when the dilatation is unsatisfactory. The hood should be retrieved after a series of interventions. It can be retrieved simply by reinserting the endoscope into the overtube that had been left in place, grasping the hood with a basket catheter (FG-33W, Olympus) under endoscopic guidance, and removing the endoscope together with the overtube (Fig. 11.4.13).

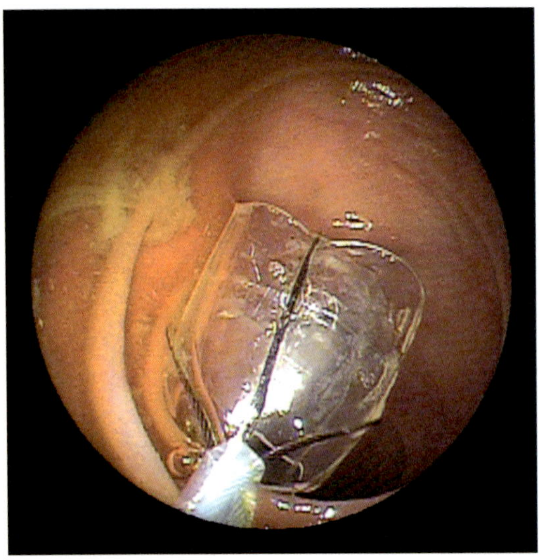

Fig. 11.4.13. Food being captured and retrieved with a basket catheter

11.4.4 Preparation of the Plastic Tube

A handmade plastic tube used for balloon dilatation is prepared by cutting a storage plastic tube of a Jagwire (0.35 mm diameter, 450 cm length) to a length of 150 cm. The tip of the plastic tube is then blunted by heating, and gold foil is placed with a tape so it can be identified under fluoroscopic guidance. The gold foil is taken from the mark at the tip of the overtube of double-balloon endoscopy (Fig. 11.4.14).

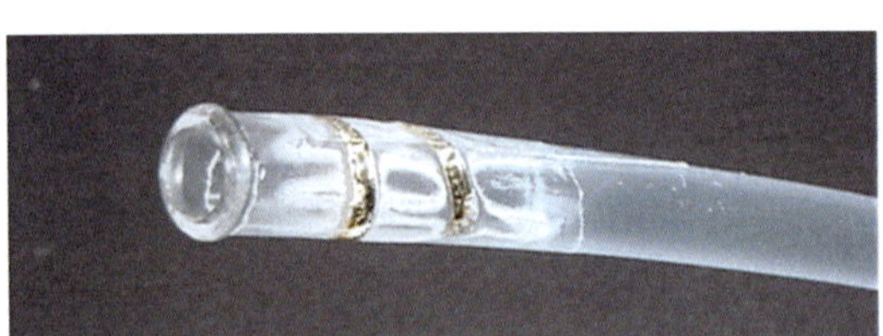

Fig. 11.4.14. Tip of a handmade plastic tube

12 Other Applications

12.1 Double-Balloon Endoscopy as Colonoscopy

12.1.1 Difficult Colonoscopy

Total colonoscopy has become common practice, and it is less frequently difficult to complete a total colonoscopy by inserting an endoscope into the cecum. In some patients, however, even skilled endoscopists give up inserting the endoscope into the cecum because of its difficulty.

As described in Chapter 5, what makes insertion of a colonoscope and other endoscopes difficult is the stretching of the intestine that has formed bends or loops. The endoscope tip does not advance because endoscope insertion is translated into stretching the intestine. Moreover, intestinal stretching causes discomfort to the patient (Fig. 12.1.1).

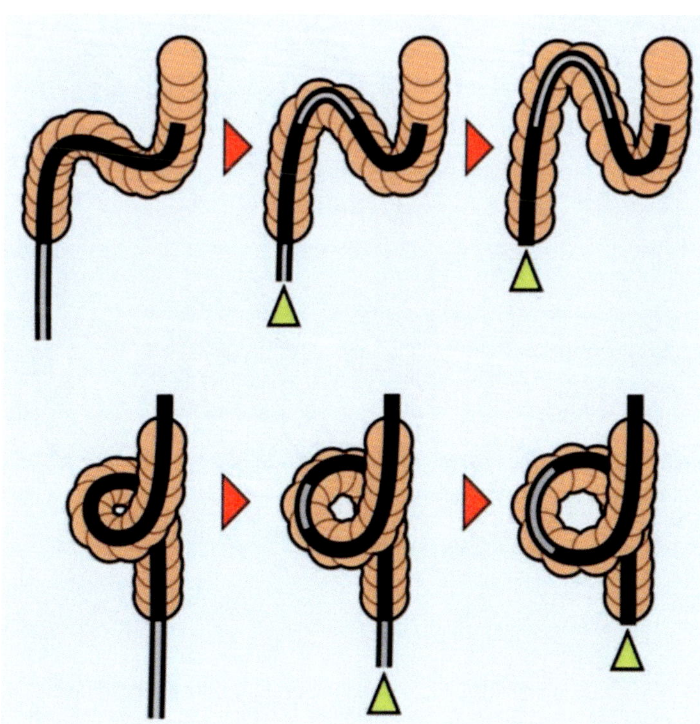

Fig. 12.1.1. Stretching of curved or looped intestine

Representative conditions that make insertion of a colonoscope difficult include adhesions in the sigmoid colon and the transverse colon. The presence of an adhesion does not necessarily mean an obstacle to colonoscopic insertion. When an adhesion complicates the anatomy, however, it makes insertion difficult.

Adhesions in the sigmoid colon often result from appendectomy, gynecologic surgery, peritonitis, and colonic diverticulum; and insertion of a colonoscope is difficult when an adhesion of the sigmoid colon to the right lower abdomen precludes straightening the sigmoid colon. The endoscope tip may be advanced into the descending colon with difficulty but not beyond the splenic flexure because the sigmoid colon is only stretched and not straightened (Fig. 12.1.2a).

Adhesions in the transverse colon are often associated with cholecystectomy, gastrectomy, or peritonitis; and colonoscope insertion is difficult when adhesion of the transverse colon to the lower abdomen precludes straightening the transverse colon. The endoscope may be advanced into the middle of the transverse colon but not beyond the hepatic flexure because the sagging transverse colon cannot be lifted up to straighten it, resulting in stretching of the transverse colon (Fig. 12.1.3a).

When adhesions in the sigmoid colon or transverse colon preclude straightening the intestine through which the double-balloon endoscope has advanced, the balloon at the tip of the overtube grips the intestine from inside, and the intestinal tract over the overtube may form a loop or bend but not stretch. For this reason, insertion of the endoscope shaft is effectively transmitted to the endoscope tip without stretching the intestine and allows deep

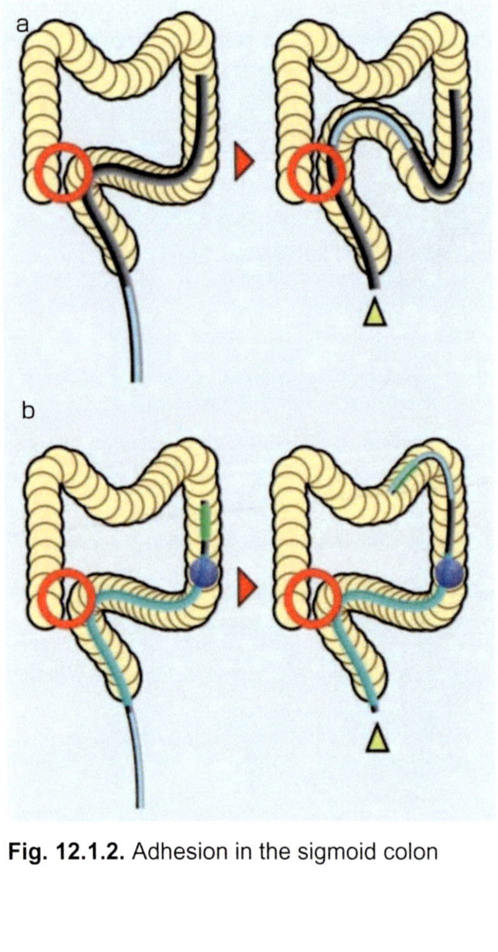

Fig. 12.1.2. Adhesion in the sigmoid colon

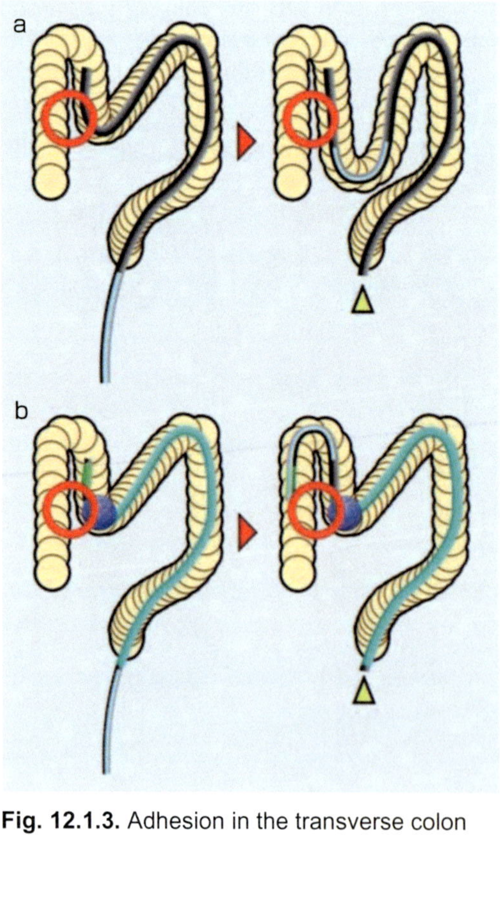

Fig. 12.1.3. Adhesion in the transverse colon

advancement of the endoscope (Figs. 12.1.2b, 12.1.3b). Inhibiting any stretching of the intestine substantially reduces the patient's discomfort.

The following is a specific method of insertion in the presence of an adhesion in the sigmoid colon (Fig. 12.1.4). First, the endoscope with a deflated balloon at the tip is inserted through the anus without specific efforts for straightening. The endoscope is advanced until further insertion is difficult (in most cases, up to the sigmoid–descending colon junction). Then the balloon at the endoscope tip is inflated to secure the endoscope, and an overtube with a balloon attached is inserted along the endoscope. After the balloons on the endoscope and the overtube are inflated, the entire endoscope is pulled back with the endoscope tip left in position. This procedure does not necessarily require straightening of the sigmoid colon. Because the overtube with the balloon prevents stretching, an angulated sigmoid colon does not interfere with the endoscope insertion. After the balloon at the endoscope tip is deflated, the endoscope is advanced again, and similar procedures are repeated before the splenic flexure and the hepatic flexure. This strategy allows the endoscope to reach the cecum without unnecessary stretching of the sigmoid colon that is impossible to straighten.

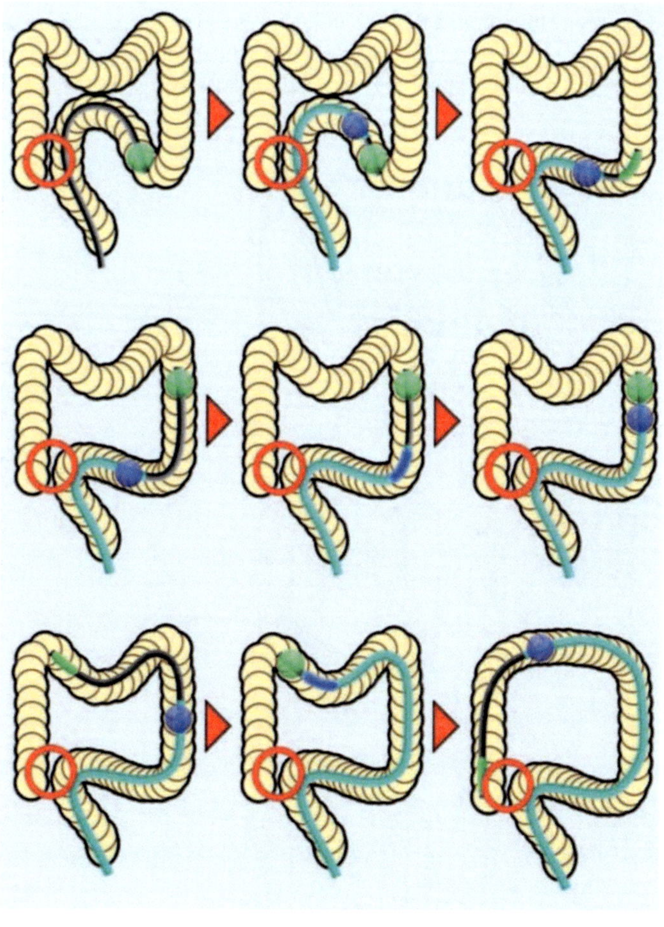

Fig. 12.1.4. Insertion in the presence of an adhesion in the sigmoid colon

The following is a specific method of insertion in the presence of adhesions in the transverse colon (Fig. 12.1.5). As described for the presence of an adhesion in the sigmoid colon, the balloon is used to insert the endoscope until it reaches the splenic flexure. After the tip of the overtube with the balloon attached is secured just before reaching the splenic flexure, the endoscope is advanced beyond the splenic flexure until further insertion is difficult. Then the balloon at the endoscope tip is inflated to secure the endoscope, and the overtube with the balloon attached is inserted along the endoscope. After both balloons (at the endoscope and the overtube) are inflated, the entire endoscope is pulled back with the endoscope tip left in position. Thereafter, the balloon at the endoscope tip is deflated, and the endoscope is further advanced. When insertion is difficult at the hepatic flexure or other locations, a similar procedure may be attempted. This strategy allows the endoscope to reach the cecum without stretching the transverse colon that is impossible to straighten.

An actual case is presented here. A 70-year-old man with previous cholecystectomy was found to have polyps in the ascending colon and the transverse colon on barium enema examination. A skilled endoscopist performed conventional colonoscopy but failed to advance the scope beyond the splenic flexure because the sigmoid colon with an adhesion was not straightened but only stretched. On another day, a second experienced endoscopist performed unsuccessful colonoscopy. The double-balloon method later allowed us to advance the endoscope beyond the splenic flexure into the transverse colon, with the sigmoid colon left angulated. Although an adhesion again precluded straightening the transverse colon, the overtube with a balloon attached was inserted into and secured in the trans-

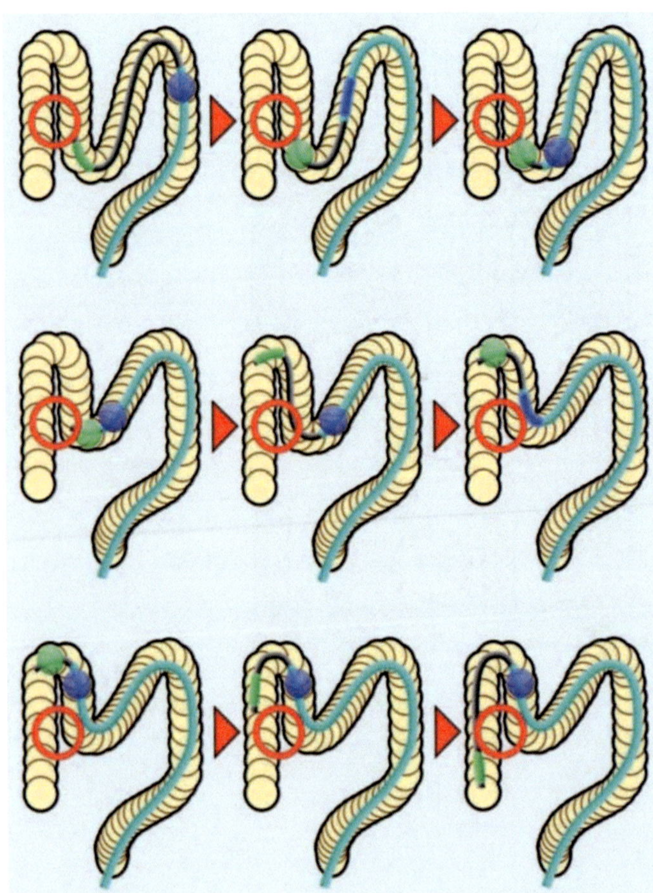

Fig. 12.1.5. Insertion in the presence of an adhesion in the transverse colon

verse colon, enabling the endoscope to advance beyond the hepatic flexure into the cecum and finally the terminal ileum (Fig. 12.1.6). The polyps in the ascending colon and the transverse colon found on barium enema were successfully resected, and the examination and treatment were completed without patient discomfort.

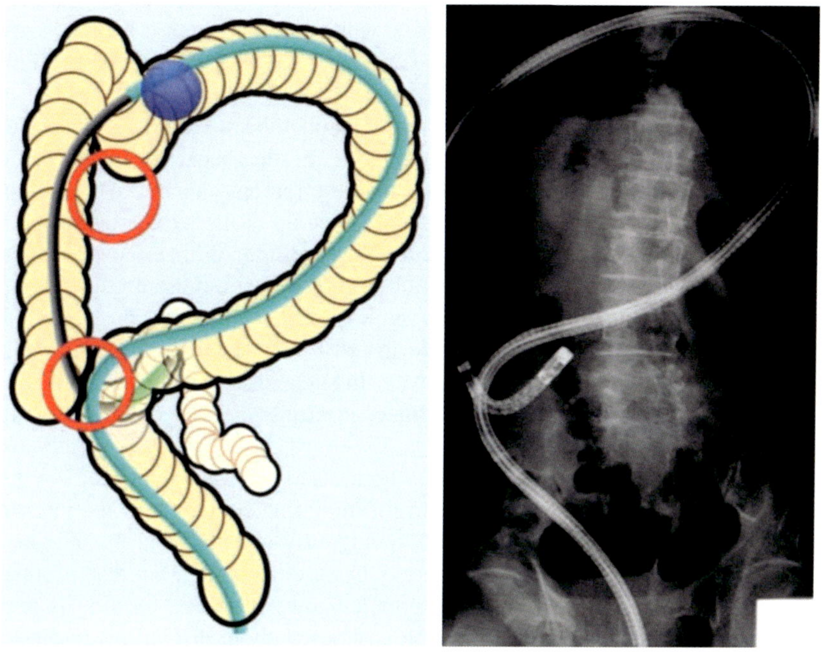

Fig. 12.1.6. A case with adhesions at the sigmoid colon and the transverse colon

12.1.2 Applications in the Large Intestine Other than Technically Difficult Cases

For endoscopic treatment in the large intestine, holding the endoscope in an ideal position is essential but sometimes difficult depending on the site of the lesion. It is particularly difficult around the hepatic flexure, splenic flexure, and sigmoid colon–descending colon junction, and its failure precludes the delicate manipulation needed for endoscopic treatment. With colonoscopy, the colonoscope is manipulated distally from fixed points, such as the anus, sigmoid colon–descending colon junction, splenic flexure, and hepatic flexure, from outside of the body. The more distant the colonoscope tip is placed from the fixed point, the more difficult is the manipulation. With double-balloon endoscopy, a stable fixed support can be established in any place by holding the intestine with the balloon at the tip of the overtube. This allows delicate manipulation and safer endoscopic treatment even in areas where the conventional endoscope is difficult to manipulate.

In the presence of multiple large polyps that cannot be suctioned through the forceps channel in the distal portion of the large intestine, it may be troublesome to collect resected specimens after endoscopic polypectomy. With conventional colonoscopy, multiple resected polyp specimens may be collected with a five-nail forceps or a net at a time. However, if it is difficult, each resected polyp specimen should be grasped with a five-nail forceps, and the endoscope should be removed for collection and then reinserted to repeat the polypectomy. With double-balloon endoscopy, the endoscope can be removed, leaving the overtube with balloon attached in the deep portion of the large intestine. Thus, the endoscope tip can be placed back into the same position of the large intestine in a few seconds through the overtube after the endoscope is removed to collect each resected specimen. When endoscopic polypectomy is performed during technically challenging colonoscopy, this characteristic provides a significant advantage together with the aforementioned improved maneuverability of the endoscope.

Decompression with a long decompression tube inserted through the anus may be required in the bowel obstruction of the large intestine because of advanced colorectal cancer. A guidewire is usually inserted through the forceps channel of the colonoscope, which has been inserted into the affected region, so the tip of the wire is placed beyond the affected region. After removing the colonoscope, a dilator is inserted along the guidewire to dilate the stenosis, followed by insertion of a long decompression tube along the guidewire through the anus. When the affected region is localized in either the transverse or ascending colon, however, it may be difficult to insert a long decompression tube through the anus because the guidewire bends on the way. In such cases, placing the overtube with balloon attached near the affected region facilitates inserting a long decompression tube through the anus (Fig. 12.1.7).

As described above, in patients in whom insertion of a colonoscope is difficult, double-balloon endoscopy is extremely useful for inhibiting stretching of the intestine, substantially reducing patient discomfort, and allowing easy insertion and manipulation of the endoscope. These advantages are useful not only for challenging, but also routine, colonoscopy. Although colonoscopy has become popular now, extensive training is required to be an endoscopist capable of performing colonoscopy without discomfort to the patient. Because of the lack of skilled endoscopists in some regions, colonoscopy causes significant discomfort to patients. Double-balloon endoscopy is expected to help resolve such problems.

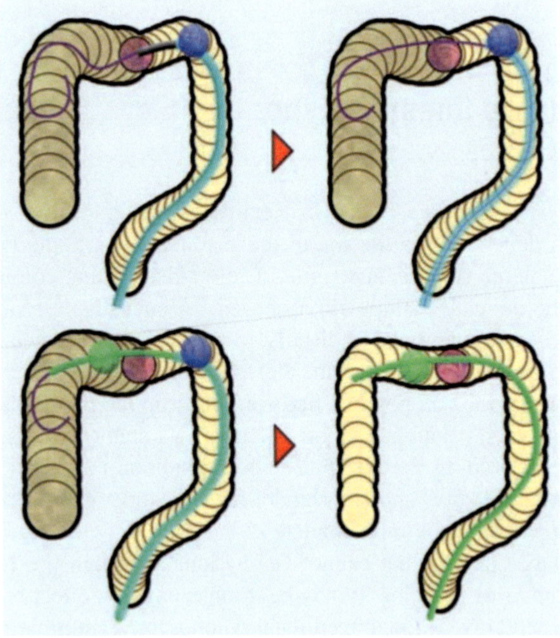

Fig. 12.1.7. Insertion of a long decompression tube through the anus

12.2 Use in Patients with Previous Intestinal Surgery

Double-balloon endoscopy allows endoscopic observation of the distal small intestine that is not accessible by conventional endoscopy. Unlike the capsule endoscope and enteroscopes inserted by the sonde method or the ropeway method that depend on peristalsis of the intestine, the double-balloon endoscope can be inserted in the direction opposite to that of intestinal peristalsis. Thus, the endoscope can be inserted into the intestinal tract reconstructed by abdominal surgery, such as the afferent loop, blind loop, and blind pouch after a Billroth II reconstruction or a Roux-en-Y reconstruction.

Not only examination but also treatment is possible, including endoscopic retrograde cholangiopancreatectomy (ERCP), via the afferent duodenal loop using lithotripsy, balloon dilatation, and stent placement; similar interventions are feasible in patients with previous choledochojejunostomy. Endoscopic treatment is feasible in patients in whom endoscopic treatment has to be ruled out because of inaccessibility using conventional techniques.

● Selection of endoscopes

As of the end of 2005, two models of double-balloon endoscopes are available: EN-450P5 with a forceps channel diameter of 2.2 mm and an outer diameter of 8.5 mm and EN-450T5 with a forceps channel diameter of 2.8 mm and an outer diameter of 9.4 mm. These scopes are used in combination with a dedicated overtube with an outer diameter of 12.2 or 13.2 mm. The two models are different in that the EN-450T5 has a thicker, more rigid endoscope shaft and a larger forceps channel, which enables the use of a variety of therapeutic devices. Because of its rigid endoscope shaft, the EN-450T5 may exhibit better insertability in patients without intraperitoneal adhesions compared with the EN-450P5; however, this property may make insertion difficult in patients with postoperative intraperitoneal adhesions. These characteristics, as well as the need for specific intervention, should be well considered when selecting an endoscope.

12.2.1 Specific Tips for Insertion in Patients with a Postoperative Intestine

Before examining patients with previous intestinal surgery, the earlier operative notes should be obtained to review the location and type of surgery. Information about the postoperative course, history of bowel obstruction, daily bowel movements, and location of the surgical incision in the abdominal wall may help estimate the degree and location of adhesions.

Adhesions may limit the mobility of the intestine in the abdomen and make insertion difficult. Such a problem can be addressed by changes in the fixed point supported with the balloon at the tip of the overtube, postural change, manual pressure, the use of a guidewire, or other techniques.

One of the characteristics of double-balloon endoscopy is the ability to manipulate the endoscope, with the balloon at the tip of the overtube as a fixed support. When insertion is difficult, a change in the position of the fixed support may improve the situation. Postural change is associated with changes in the weight-bearing part, the positional relation between the intestine and the endoscope in the abdominal cavity, and the distribution of intestinal contents, thereby resolving the deadlock. As in the case of a long decompression tube insertion, one of the tips for abdominal maneuvering is to apply pressure on regions so a redundant loop of the endoscope is reduced. The abdominal wall around the endoscope tip may be pressed or tapped, which allows the endoscope tip to advance.

When a guidewire is used, care should be taken to avoid intestinal perforation by the guidewire. Thus, a soft-tipped guidewire is inserted and advanced through the forceps channel, followed by endoscope insertion. If the direction of the lumen is unclear during insertion of the guidewire, inflating the balloon at the endoscope tip and injecting a contrast agent into the forceps channel allows selective contrast enhancement of the lumen ahead, which helps with guidewire insertion.

Insertion into a bypassed intestine requires identification of the anastomotic site. Because of insertion with minimal air insufflation, the anastomotic site may be missed during insertion of the endoscope and identified only during its withdrawal. To reduce the examination time, it is necessary to collect detailed information and approximate the location of the anastomotic site before examination.

To identify the anastomotic site, attention should be paid to discontinuity and fusion of Kerckring's folds, luminal dilatation, direction of peristalsis, and quantity of bile. With a Roux-en-Y anastomosis, bile flows into the intestinal tract from the afferent loop; therefore, the amount of bile increases when the endoscope advances beyond the anastomotic site. In addition, the intestinal tract dilates and Kerckring's folds fuse at the anastomotic site, points that are useful for identification. Peristalsis in the efferent loop and antiperistalsis in the afferent loop help determine the position of the endoscope.

The secret for successful insertion into the bypassed intestine beyond the anastomotic site is to reduce the angle at the anastomotic site as much as possible. The angle can be reduced by pulling or pushing the endoscope, depending on the patient (Fig. 12.2.1). Even when the endoscope tip is advanced beyond the anastomotic site, it is often difficult to manipulate the endoscope reliably until the balloon at the tip of the overtube is secured in a place beyond the anastomotic site. When insertion is difficult, it is strongly recommended that the balloon at the endoscope tip be inflated and secured to advance the tip of the overtube beyond the anastomotic site.

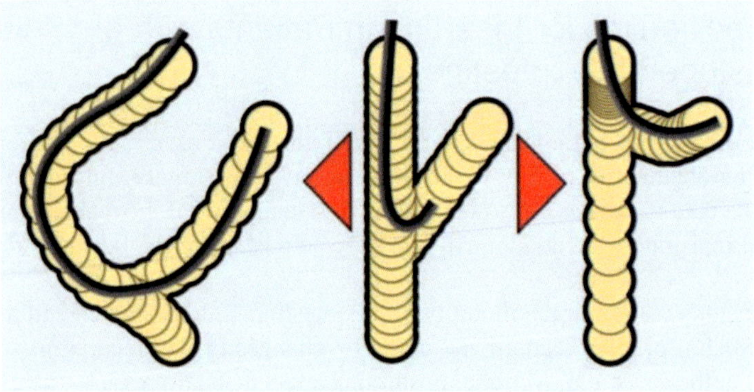

Fig. 12.2.1. Procedure to reduce the angle at the anastomotic site

When the endoscope is advanced into the afferent loop of a Billroth II reconstruction or a Roux-en-Y reconstruction for endoscopic intervention, instruments should be inserted through the forceps channel for manipulation. The double-balloon endoscopes EN-450P5 and EN-450T5, available as of the end of 2005, have forceps channel diameters of 2.2 and 2.8 mm, respectively. The use of therapeutic devices is limited by the forceps channel diameter and the working length, which is as long as 200 cm. To address the limitation, the double-balloon endoscope inserted into a region of interest may be replaced with another endoscope that has a larger forceps channel diameter and shorter working length while the overtube is securely anchored with the balloon. The use of a shorter overtube instead of the 145-cm standard balloon-attached overtube allows the use of an endoscope with a shorter working length so long as it is thin enough to pass through the overtube, thereby offering a wide choice of endoscopes and therapeutic devices for use during endoscopic interventions.

As an example, we present a case of endoscopic mucosal resection (EMR) of duodenal cancer in the afferent duodenal loop after Roux-en-Y reconstruction. At that time, the EN-450T5 was not commercially available, and the EN-450P5 with a forceps channel diameter of 2.2 mm was used. First, the overtube with a balloon attached, TS-12140, was modified to have a shorter length of 70 cm, and the double-balloon endoscope was inserted into the blind end of the afferent duodenal loop. Then the tip of the overtube with a balloon attached was advanced into the afferent duodenal loop, and the balloon at the tip of the overtube was inflated to secure the overtube. The endoscope was removed with the balloon-attached overtube left in place, and the endoscope GIF-XQ240 (outer diameter 9.0 mm, forceps channel diameter 2.8 mm) (Olympus) was inserted to perform EMR (Fig. 12.2.2) (see section 11.3.5).

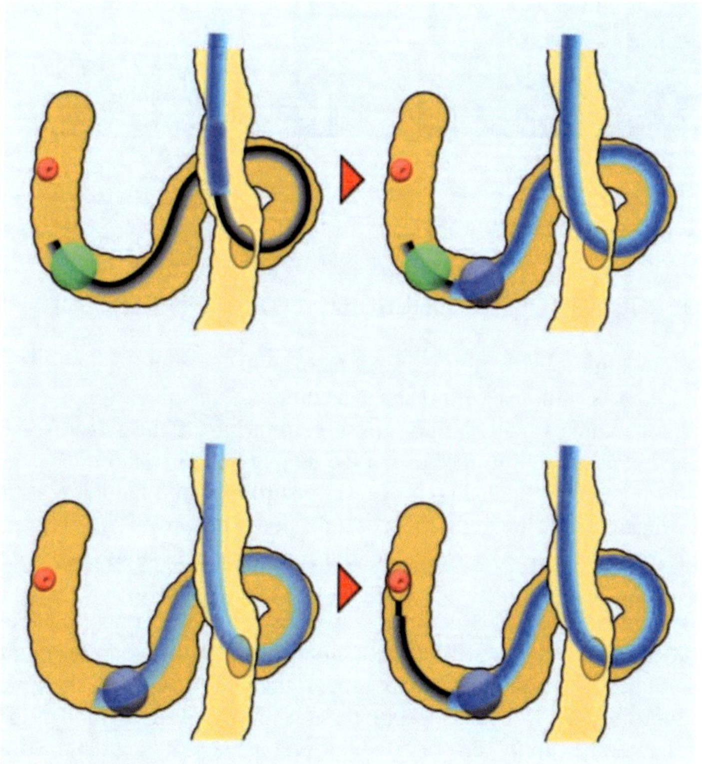

Fig. 12.2.2. Endoscopic mucosal resection in the afferent duodenal loop

A similar method may be used to perform ERCP, endoscopic papillary balloon dilation (EPBD), lithotripsy, or tube stent placement for the treatment of choledocholithiasis after Roux-en-Y reconstruction. The procedure is applicable in other clinical settings as well.

In patients without a duodenal papilla after choledochojejunostomy, cholangiography can be performed by injecting a contrast agent into the forceps channel with the balloon at the double-balloon endoscope tip inflated (Fig. 12.2.3).

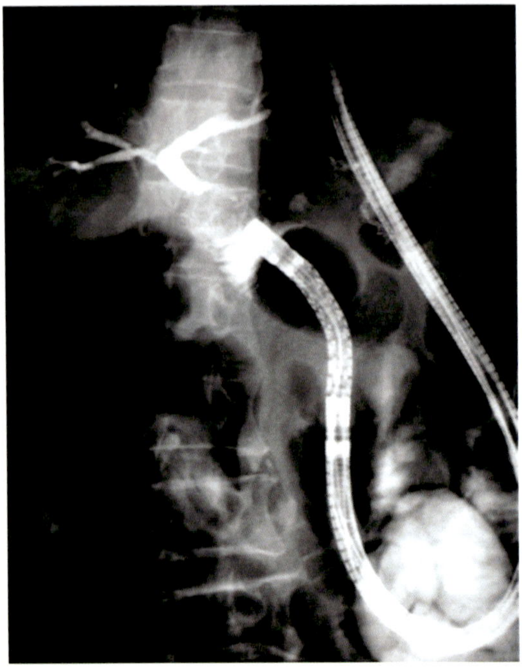

Fig. 12.2.3. Cholangiography in a patient with previous choledochojejunostomy

12.2.2 Investigation of the Cause of Bowel Obstruction

Adhesive intestinal obstruction may occur in patients with previous abdominal surgery. Contrast-enhanced studies with a long decompression tube, computed tomography, and magnetic resonance imaging may allow estimation of the site responsible for bowel obstruction but not tattooing. The use of the double-balloon endoscope enables exact identification of the region responsible for bowel obstruction and tattooing at the site. Tattooing facilitates laparoscopic identification of adhesions responsible for bowel obstruction and allows minimally invasive laparoscopic division of the adhesions. Laparoscopic visibility is increased by placing tattoos on the opposite sides of the lumen.

In patients with bowel obstruction undergoing decompression with a long decompression tube, inserting the overtube with a balloon attached, with a long decompression tube as a guide, facilitates insertion of the endoscope to the region at which the tip of a long decompression tube is placed (a long decompression tube-guiding method). Specifically, a long decompression tube (up to 16F) inserted through the nostril is cut at the proximal connector and withdrawn through the mouth. During this procedure it is desirable to keep the balloon at the tip of a long decompression tube inflated. After a guidewire is inserted through a long decompression tube to reduce loops, the balloon-attached overtube for double-balloon endoscopy is inserted along a long decompression tube. The overtube is inserted to the tip of a long decompression tube, and then the balloon at the tip of the overtube is inflated and held in place. Subsequently, the balloon at the tip of a long decompression tube is deflated, and a long decompression tube and guidewire are removed; the overtube with a balloon attached is left in place. Within a few seconds, the endoscope can be passed through the overtube to its tip, where the tip of a long decompression tube was previously positioned (Fig. 12.2.4).

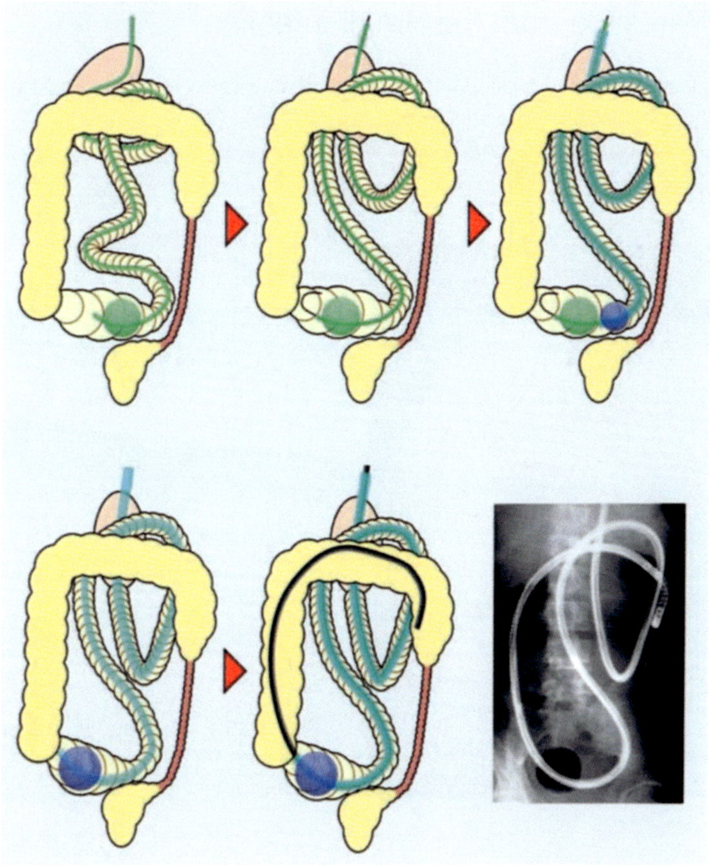

Fig. 12.2.4. A long decompression tube guiding method

References

1. Kuno A, Yamamoto H, Kita H, et al (2004) Application of double-balloon enteroscopy through Roux-en-Y anastomosis for the endoscopic mucosal resection of an early carcinoma in the duodenal afferent limb. Gastrointest Endosc 60:1032–1034
2. Yano T, Yamamoto H, Kita H, et al. (2005) Technical modification of the double-balloon endoscopy to access the proximal side of the stenosis in the distal colon: report of a case. Gastrointest Endosc 62:302–304

12.3 Removal of Foreign Bodies from the Small Intestine

The double-balloon endoscope can be inserted into the entire small intestine and a bypassed intestinal tract for the purpose of examination. With a therapeutic device, it allows removal of foreign bodies from the small intestine.

12.3.1 Removal of Parasites from the Small Intestine

Double-balloon endoscopy revealed a parasite in the small intestine (Ascaris). It was successfully removed endoscopically from the body (Fig. 12.3.1) (kindly provided by Dr. Zhong Jie, Ruijin Hospital, Shanghai Second Medical University, China).

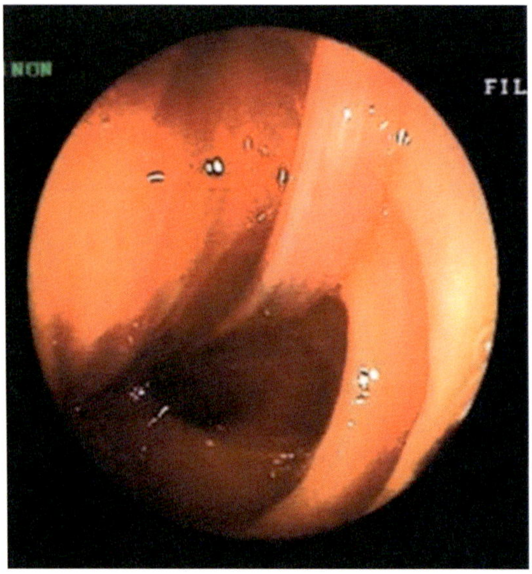

Fig. 12.3.1. Parasite in the small intestine found by double-balloon endoscopy

12.3.2 Removal of Capsule Endoscope

Because of retention of a capsule endoscope in a stenotic region of the small intestine, the double-balloon endoscope was inserted through the mouth, which allowed direct identification of the capsule endoscope rostral to the stenotic region (Fig. 12.3.2). Through the forceps channel of the endoscope, a Roth Net modified to have a longer sheath length (net size 25 mm) (US Endoscopy Group, Mentor, OH, USA) was used to hold the capsule endoscope to remove it from the body (Fig. 12.3.3) (kindly provided by Dr. Shu Tanaka, Third Department of Internal Medicine, Nippon Medical School, Japan). When the treatment-type double-balloon endoscope EN-450T5 is used, a Roth Net compatible with a 3.2-mm channel with a net size of 40 mm can be modified to have a thin profile to be applicable.

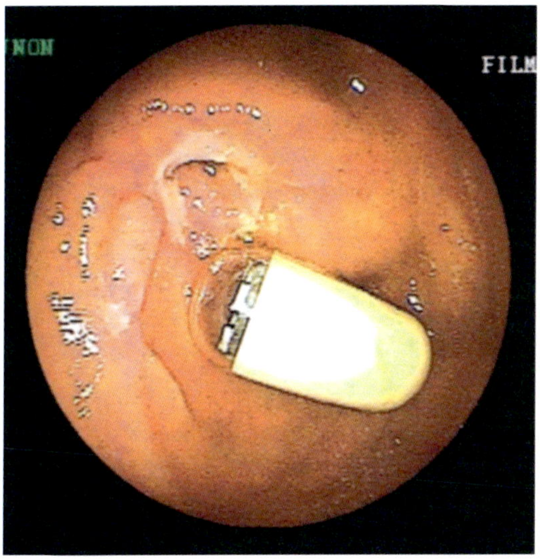

Fig. 12.3.2. Capsule endoscope retained rostral to the stenotic site

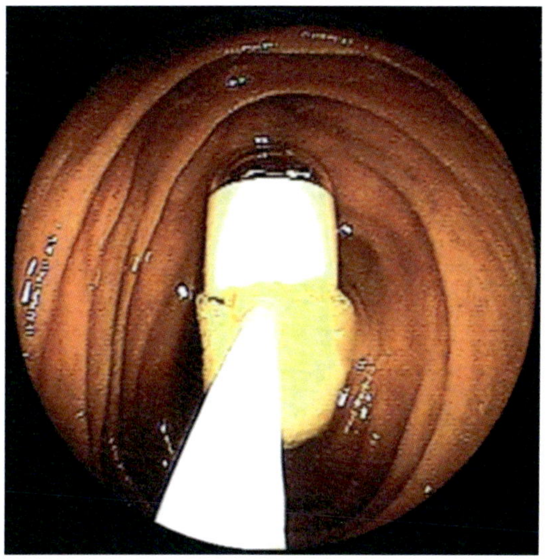

Fig.12.3.3. Capsule retrieved with a modified Roth Net with a longer sheath length

Subject Index

A

B

C

D

E

Kolibri 360 GmbH
Ferdinand-Jühlke-Straße 7
99095 Erfurt, Deutschland
produktsicherheit@kolibri360.de